ABNORMALITIES OF COMPANION ANIMALS:

Analysis of Heritability

ABNORMALITIES OF COMPANION ANIMALS:

Analysis of Heritability

C. W. Foley
J. F. Lasley
G. D. Osweiler

The Iowa State University Press, **AMES,** *Iowa*

CHARLES W. FOLEY, Professor of Veterinary Anatomy and Physiology at the University of Missouri, has specialized in physiological genetics and endocrinology and reproduction. He has held teaching and research posts at Purdue University, the University of Georgia, and the University of Missouri. He is coeditor of *The Oviduct and Its Functions.* He received the B.S., M.S., and Ph.D. degrees from the University of Missouri.

JOHN F. LASLEY is Professor and Chairman of the Department of Animal Husbandry at the University of Missouri. He has conducted research in both physiology and genetics of farm animals and is author or coauthor of numerous scientific and popular articles in these areas. Dr. Lasley is the author of *Genetics of Livestock Improvement* and coauthor (with Dr. J. R. Campbell) of *The Science of Animals That Serve Mankind.* He has taught thousands of college students and has received several awards for research and teaching. In 1968 he received the Distinguished Teacher Award from the American Society of Animal Science, and in 1978 he received the Outstanding Faculty Award in Agriculture at the University of Missouri. He has presented many lectures on genetics of livestock improvement in the United States and foreign countries.

GARY D. OSWEILER has specialized in pathology and toxicology with additional experience in clinical medicine. He has been affiliated with Veterinary Diagnostic Laboratories at Iowa State University and the University of Missouri with teaching responsibilities in toxicology and diagnostic pathology. He is a diplomate in the American Board of Veterinary Toxicology and is coauthor of a textbook in veterinary toxicology. He received the D.V.M., M.S., and Ph.D. degrees from Iowa State University.

© 1979 The Iowa State University Press
All rights reserved

Composed and printed by
The Iowa State University Press
Ames, Iowa 50010

First edition, 1979

Library of Congress Cataloging in Publication Data

Foley, C   W
    Abnormalities of companion animals.

    Includes bibliographies and index.
    1. Veterinary genetics. 2. Dogs—Diseases—Genetic aspects. 3. Cats—Diseases—Genetic aspects. 4. Horses—Diseases—Genetic aspects. I. Lasley, John Foster, 1913-   joint author. II.   Osweiler, G. D., 1942-   joint author. III. Title.
SF756.5.F64   636.089'6'042   78-31919
ISBN 0-8138-0940-1

CONTENTS

PREFACE

Each year more and more abnormalities of structure and function of companion animals are reported in the literature. Some of these abnormalities are congenital, that is, they are present at birth. Pups, kittens, or foals are born with structural or functional disorders. Congenital defects may or may not be inherited. Some abnormalities are not congenital. These noncongenital defects are not present at birth, but their effects appear later in the animal's life. These noncongenital defects also may or may not be inherited.

To provide the necessary information to animal breeders, the practicing veterinarian needs to be able to recognize an inherited condition or defect and should understand the mode of inheritance of the defect in order to suggest a workable solution for clients to eliminate the undesirable characteristics from their breeding programs so as to prevent long-term serious effects to the breed concerned. Likewise, the breeder needs to understand the defect to be able to work with the veterinarian in the elimination of the trait.

The material presented here is intended to outline the fundamental principles of animal genetics in such a manner that it will be useful to the veterinarian and animal breeders in detecting genetic defects. It will assemble in one place and, it is hoped, present in appropriate depth and breadth basic information concerning the inheritance of most common genetic defects and conditions observed in companion animals, the pathophysiologic basis behind the inheritance of these anomalies, and recommendations to the breeder. Lists of selected references are given for further study.

This material is in no way intended to suggest that every defect has a genetic base. However, all defects discussed in this manuscript were considered by the original researchers to have a genetic or possible genetic base. In many cases too few animals or experiments were available for firm conclusions.

For certain disorders the majority of published information is from one laboratory; for other defects a variety of sources has been used.

PART I

Introduction

CHAPTER 1

Fundamental Principles of Genetics

All life comes from preexisting life. Among the mammals, the newborn individual must have a father and a mother. The offspring resembles each parent in many ways because it receives approximately one-half its inheritance from each of them. How this is done constitutes the science of genetics.

Genes are the smallest units of inheritance and they are responsible, in a general way, for the form and function of each individual. This is true because genes control the thousands of biochemical reactions within the animal's body. Thus the proper function of the body is dependent on the proper function of each of the thousands of genes in body cells. Each gene has a particular function to perform. A change in a gene (a mutation) so that it no longer performs a certain function is responsible in many instances for the occurrence of defects of anatomy and physiology in newborn individuals.

It is the purpose here to briefly present the nature of genes, how they function, and how they may be related to the form and function of the individual.

THE CELL AND ITS COMPONENTS

The body of each animal is made up of billions of minute building blocks called cells. Each animal begins life as a single cell, resulting from the union of the sperm and egg in the process of fertilization.

The body of each animal contains cells of which most have a cell membrane, a nucleus, and cytoplasm. Within the cytoplasm, which may vary

3

widely in size and shape, are many units called "organelles," each of which has some basic function in the life and/or reproduction of the cell. A diagram of a cell (Fig. 1.1) shows some of these organelles in the cytoplasm. The *ribosomes* in the cytoplasm are responsible for manufacturing many different kinds of proteins. Many *Golgi bodies* are also found in the cytoplasm and they are thought to be the site of the synthesis of large carbohydrate molecules that perform certain vital functions in the body. *Mitochondria* are the sites of chemical reactions supplying energy for various reactions in the cells. *Lysosomes* are small bodies in the cytoplasm containing digestive enzymes that break down all the major constituents of living organisms. Abnormal lysosomes are known to be involved in certain diseases of humans.

The nucleus is the "director" of synthesis of the cell or of the activities of the organelles, etc., and contains threadlike structures called chromosomes (*chromo* meaning color; *soma* meaning body).

The Chromosomes

The hereditary material, the genes, are carried on the chromosomes. Each chromosome contains many genes along its length and may be de-

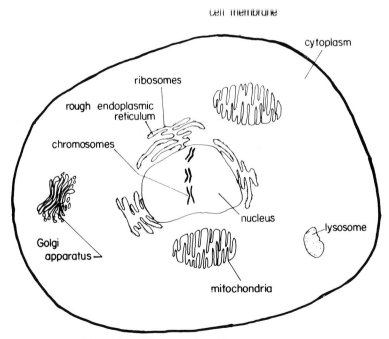

Fig. 1.1. *Diagram of a cell.*

scribed as being similar to a long string of beads with each bead being a gene. Each species of animal normally has a characteristic number of chromosomes. Normal chromosome numbers for some common species are listed in Table 1.1. Chromosomes occur in pairs in all body cells that possess a nucleus except the gametes (ova and sperm) where they occur in half pairs. These pairs of chromosomes are *homologous chromosomes* (*homo* meaning alike; *logous* meaning structure). One of the pairs of chromosomes is known as the *sex chromosomes* because this pair determines the sex of the individual. In mammals the female possesses two X chromosomes in each body cell, whereas the male possesses an X and a Y. The X chromosome is considerably longer than the Y and therefore carries more genetic material (Fig. 1.2). In poultry the sex chromosomes are called X and W (or sometimes Z and W), with the X chromosome the larger of the two. The female is ZW and the male XX, which is exactly opposite of what is found in mammals. All the chromosomes other than the sex chromosomes are called *autosomes*. Thus an autosomal recessive gene is one carried on the autosomes; a sex-linked recessive gene is one carried on the X or Y chromosome (Fig. 1.3).

Of each pair of chromosomes (the 2n number), one normally comes from the individual's father and the other from its mother, although in the case of fatherless turkeys both chromosomes of each pair come from the mother. A parent normally transmits one chromosome of each pair, not both, to any one offspring through the sperm or egg, with chance determining which one of the pair will be transmitted from the parent to a given offspring. When the egg is fertilized by the spermatozoa, the pairs of chromosomes in each body cell of the new individual are restored to the normal 2n number for that species.

Table 1.1. Normal chromosome numbers for some selected species of animals

Species	Normal 2n Number
Domestic horse *(Equus caballus)*	64
Domestic pig *(Sus scrofa)*	38
Domestic cattle *(Bos taurus)*	60
Domestic cattle *(Bos indica)*	60
American bison *(Bison bison)*	60
Domestic sheep *(Ovis aries)*	54
Domestic dog *(Canis familiaris)*	78
Domestic goat *(Capra hircus)*	60
Donkey *(Equus asinus)*	62
Domestic fowl *(Gallus domesticus)*	78
Man *(Homo sapiens)*	46
Domestic cat *(Felis catus)*	38
Laboratory rabbit *(Oryctolagus cuniculus)*	44
Chinese hamster *(Cricetulus griseus)*	22
Golden hamster *(Mesocricetus auratus)*	44
Mouse *(Mus musculus)*	40
Rat *(Rattus norvegicus)*	42

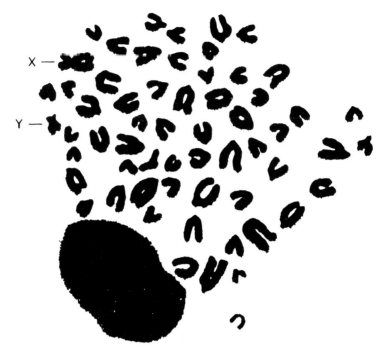

Fig 1 7 *The chromosome complement of the bovine showing the X and the Y chromosomes of the male. These chromosomes were from a culture of lymphocytes from the blood. The large, dark object in the lower left-hand portion of the picture is a lymphocyte just beginning to divide. When chromosomes can be stained and photographed, each chromosome has divided but the two parts are still attached at the centromere. The length of the chromosome and the attachment helps identify certain pairs of chromosomes in the body cells.*

Abnormal Chromosomes

Chromosome numbers are generally held constant within a species from one generation to another, but occasionally chromosome abnormalities, called aberrations, occur. When they occur they are usually detrimental to the individual and may even cause its death (lethal). Abnormalities include those due to numbers of chromosomes, those due to improper structure, and those due to mixtures of cell types.

NUMERICAL ABNORMALITIES. Abnormalities of chromosome numbers are of two general types. The first, known as *polyploidy* (or euploidy), involves a duplication of complete sets of chromosomes. Instead of the normal pairs that are diploid, or 2n, the individual may possessess 3n, 4n, or possibly more. In mammals, the duplication of entire sets of chromosomes appears

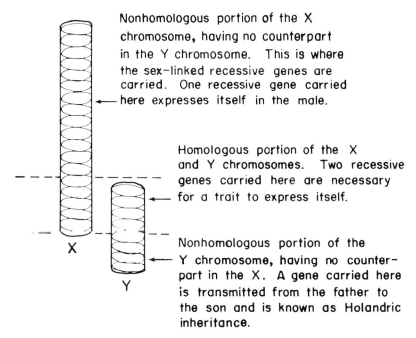

Nonhomologous portion of the X chromosome, having no counterpart in the Y chromosome. This is where the sex-linked recessive genes are carried. One recessive gene carried here expresses itself in the male.

Homologous portion of the X and Y chromosomes. Two recessive genes carried here are necessary for a trait to express itself.

Nonhomologous portion of the Y chromosome, having no counterpart in the X. A gene carried here is transmitted from the father to the son and is known as Holandric inheritance.

Fig. 1.3. *A drawing representing the X and Y chromosome complement in male animals.*

to be lethal, whereas in plants such individuals are sometimes viable. Some spontaneous abortions in humans are due to the polyploid condition. The second numerical abnormality in chromosome numbers is known as *aneuploidy,* where a single chromosome or a limited number of chromosomes is involved. The individual may possess one more chromosome than normal (2n + 1) or may lack one chromosome (2n − 1). Two or more chromosomes may be involved instead of one, which would result in either the 2n + 2 or the 2n − 2 condition. Mongolism in humans is due to an extra chromosome or a part of an extra chromosome. Other abnormalities of this kind involve other chromosome pairs in the human body cells.

Aneuploidy involving the sex chromosomes occurs quite often in both humans and farm animals, but it has been studied in more detail in humans. About 1 in 400 births in humans involves sex chromosome abnormalities. Such abnormalities can involve a condition of XXY or XYY. Some XXXY individuals have also been described. Other individuals are known to possess only one X and no Y (XO). Individuals possessing no sex chromosomes (OO) have not been described, probably because such a condition would be lethal very early in embryonic development.

STRUCTURAL ABNORMALITIES. Several structural chromosome abnormalities have been described in the scientific literature, and most of these also are detrimental or lethal

The structural abnormality known as a *translocation* is one in which a portion of a chromosome is broken off from one chromosome and becomes attached to the end of another not homologous to it. This is harmful to the individual in some cases but not in others.

A *deletion* is a chromosome abnormality in which a part of a chromosome is missing (deleted). It is usually harmful and often lethal in the affected individual.

A *duplication* means that a part of a chromosome is replicated or duplicated. For example, in meiosis the homologous chromosomes come together (synapse) and then separate again in later cell division. At times a part of one chromosome may break and remain attached to its homologous partner during synapsis, resulting in a duplication of chromosomal material and genes in that individual. A duplication may also have harmful effects.

The normal arrangement of the genes on the chromosome may be changed, resulting in an *inversion* of their order on the chromosome. To illustrate an inversion let us assume that the normal sequence of genes on a chromosome is $\overline{a\ b\ c\ d\ e}$ f. Breakage and the reunion of the same chromosome parts may result in a new sequence of genes such as $\overline{a\ b\ d\ c\ e}$ f in which the order of c and d is reversed or inverted.

Isochromosomes also have been observed in the study of chromosomes. In cell division each chromosome forms two sister chromatids bound together at one point by the centromere. Normally, the splitting of the sister chromatids occurs longitudinally, but it may occur in a transverse manner, resulting in two chromosomes that have equal arms but are unlike genetically, as shown in Figure 1.4. Other structural chromosome abnormalities include broken chromosomes and ring chromosomes. The ring chromosome is illustrated in Figure 1.5.

MIXED CELL TYPES. Abnormalities of this kind include *chimerism* and *mosaicism*. Chimerism is a condition in which one individual may possess a chromosome complement from two different sources or genotypes. For example, a heifer born twin with a bull calf is called a freemartin and is almost always sterile. Her white blood cells, and possibly other cells of the body, have some cells from her own body that possess XX chromosomes and others from her twin brother that possess XY chromosomes. She has some XY chromosomes from her brother apparently because they had a common blood supply during intrauterine life. Some scientists have been able to fuse two different fertilized mouse eggs that develop normally to produce a single mouse with chromosomes from two different genetic sources. This is also an example of chimerism.

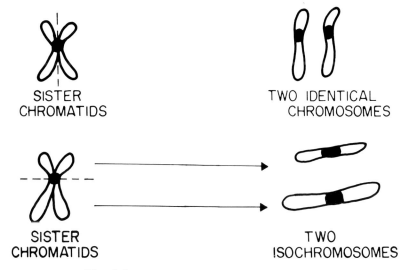

Fig. 1.4.

Mosaicism occurs in an individual where some cells may possess the 2n number of chromosomes and others the 3n number. All sources of chromosomes, however, are from that one individual or one genotype.

Chromosome abnormalities may occur naturally, but others may be induced by exposure to drugs, X-rays, and possibly certain chemicals in the diet.

CELL DIVISION

Cells increase in number by undergoing division. Two general types of cell division are known. These are *mitosis* and *meiosis*. Mitosis is the type of cell division in which the new cells produced (daughter cells) are duplicates

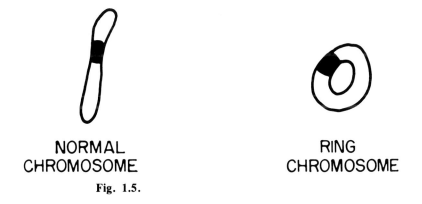

Fig. 1.5.

of the original mother cell, with all possessing the 2n (diploid) number of chromosomes. Meiosis is cell division in the gonads (ovary or testes) in which the 2n number of chromosomes is reduced to the 1n, or haploid, number in the sex cells. This reduction in chromosome number is necessary so that the union of the sperm and egg at fertilization will restore the normal 2n number of chromosomes coming from each of the two parents. As shown previously, the failure to maintain the normal 2n number of chromosomes from one generation to another would result in the extinction of that species.

THE GENE AND HOW IT FUNCTIONS

A gene may be defined as a portion of DNA molecule. DNA is an abbreviation for deoxyribonucleic acid. DNA consists of a long molecule extending the length of the chromosome and resembling a long twisted ladder, although it is extremely small, being ultramicroscopic in size. The two strands of the DNA molecule, which may be compared to the two sides of a ladder, are joined together by rungs that are actually two bases of the combination A to T (adenine to thymine) or G to C (guanine to cytosine) (Fig. 1.6). Adenine always joins with thymine and guanine with cytosine. Each strand of the DNA molecule is made up of repeated units known as *nucleotides*. A nucleotide is composed of a nitrogenous base (either a purine or a pyrimidine) linked to a sugar (deoxyribose) that is also linked to a phosphoric acid molecule. DNA is found almost entirely in the nucleus of the cell. The average gene, sometimes called a *cistron,* is thought to be a portion of a double-stranded DNA molecule consisting of about 600 consecutive base pairs. Hundreds, and even thousands, of genes may be located on a single chromosome.

Genes have at least three basic functions. They reproduce themselves, they produce RNA, and they send the code to the cytoplasm of the cell for the synthesis of a specific protein.

How genes duplicate themselves is illustrated in Figure 1.7. In duplication the two strands of the DNA molecule separate at the union of the base pairs, and each strand then serves as a template, or mold, to assemble another strand to form exact duplicates of a double-stranded DNA molecule. The success of this duplication process is assured, fundamentally, by the fact that (A) always joins with (T) and (C) with (G). When each double strand separates at the base pairs, new molecules of the bases, sugar, and phosphoric acid are assembled from the cell constitutents to form two new duplicate double strands of DNA that are exactly alike.

The DNA molecule also produces molecules of RNA, which is an abbreviation for ribonucleic acid. An RNA molecule differs from a DNA molecule by containing the sugar, ribose, instead of deoxyribose. The RNA

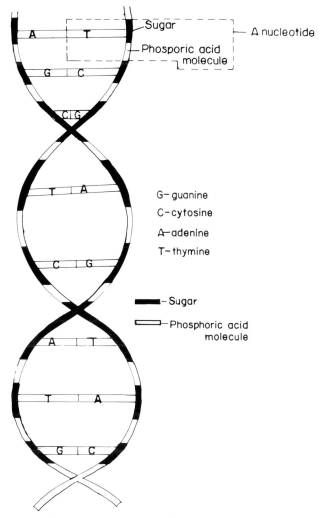

Fig. 1.6. *Diagrammatic sketch of a DNA molecule. A, T, C, and G are bases, with A always joined to T and C to G.*

molecule also differs from the DNA molecule in that it contains the base, uracil (U), which replaces thymine (T) found in DNA. In RNA, uracil always unites with adenine and guanine with cytosine. Probably most RNA molecules are formed in the nucleus in a process similar to that which produces new DNA molecules. The DNA molecule separates and one of the strands serves as a template or mold to form a single strand of RNA with (U to A) and (G to C) from cell constitutents. At least three RNA molecules are known. These are messenger RNA (mRNA), transfer RNA (tRNA), and

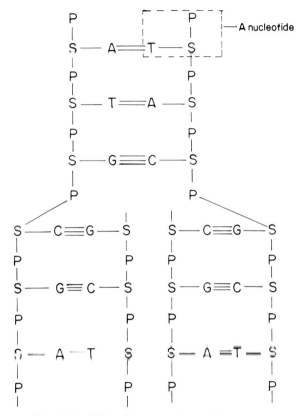

Fig. 1.7. *This illustrates how the DNA molecule exactly duplicates itself. The double-stranded DNA separates into two single strands which then assemble other parts to form two double-stranded DNA molecules that are exact duplicates of each other.*

ribosomal RNA (rRNA). These three RNA molecules are different in structure and probably perform separate functions in assembling proteins in the cytoplasm.

Another major function of the DNA molecule is to direct the synthesis of specific proteins by ribosomes in the cytoplasm of the cell. The DNA molecule sends the code to the ribosomes by means of mRNA for building a specific protein. Proteins differ from each other in the kind, number, and arrangement of the 20 amino acids found in natural proteins. Single-stranded mRNA transmits the code received from the DNA molecule in the nucleus for building proteins to the ribosomes in groups of three consecutive bases known as triplets, or codons. A codon such as UUG, for example, specifies a particular amino acid, whereas another codon such as

GGU specifies another. However, some codons may specify the same amino acid, others may not code for any amino acid at all, while still others may specify the beginning and/or ending of a chain of amino acids. This arrangement is necessary because there are 64 possible codons but only 20 amino acids.

A change in the genetic code (called a mutation) will result in a different sequence of amino acids being assembled and thus form a different protein from that produced before the mutation took place. New mutations are responsible for many recessive defects observed in animals.

CONTROL OF GENE FUNCTION

All genes within a cell are not functional. Some may function in one cell but not in another. Some may function at one time during life but not at another time. The mechanisms responsible for genes functioning, or not functioning, have been the object of research for many years. Much of the research has been done with microorganisms, and the results may not be entirely applicable to larger animals.

The theory of gene function in microorganisms proposes that there are two principal kinds of genes: the *structural genes* responsible for the synthesis of the different kinds of proteins, and the *control genes* which regulate the activity of structural genes but are not directly involved in protein synthesis. They do control protein synthesis indirectly, however, through the structural genes.

Control genes are of two kinds: the operator and the regulator genes. Operator genes appear to be located on the same chromosome as structural genes and adjacent to them. An operator gene may control the activity of one or more structural genes, turning them on and off, like a switch. Most regulator genes appear to be located on a different chromosome from structural genes although some may be located on the same chromosome. The regulator gene seems to produce a substance known as a repressor, usually a protein, which blocks the action of the operator gene, which in turn does not allow the structural genes to produce proteins because they cannot produce mRNA. A substance called an inducer (or depressor), which is usually a substrate, or a hormone, converts the repressor substance into an inactive compound, allowing the operator gene to function and the structural genes to synthesize proteins.

TRANSMISSION OF GENES FROM ONE GENERATION TO ANOTHER

Each animal receives a random one-half of its genes from each parent. This occurs because of the segregation of genes from the parents into the gametes and their recombination in the newly fertilized egg from which the new individual develops. This is brought about in nature by a particular kind of cell division called *meiosis* in the sex cells and the maintenance of the 2n number of chromosomes from each species for generation after generation because of the union of the sperm and egg in fertilization. Since the genes are carried on the chromosomes, they also occur in pairs in body cells and in half pairs in the gametes. Possible exceptions to this are sex-linked inherited traits, which will be discussed later, and where chromosome abnormalities occur.

Segregation of Genes in the Gametes—One Pair of Genes

We will use a single pair of genes carried on one pair of homologous chromosomes to illustrate how genes segregate from the primary sex cells into the gametes. A pair of genes (both influencing the same trait) such as (A) and (a) are known as *alleles,* or *allelomorphs.* With two alleles of this kind, they may combine in three different genotyes (genetic combinations); namely, AA, Aa, and aa.

An individual of genotype AA can transmit only an (A) gene through its gametes to its offspring because that is the only kind of gene it possesses in that pair. Likewise, an individual of genotype aa transmits only an (a) gene to its offspring for the same reason. This assumes, of course, that no new mutation occurs in these genes. The situation is a little different for the individual of the genotype Aa. Since it possesses both gene (A) and gene (a) it can transmit one or the other of these genes, but not both at the same time, through the sex cells to an offspring. The probability it will transmit the (A) gene to an offspring is ½ and the same probability is true for the transmission of the (a) gene to a particular offspring.

Segregation of Genes in the Gametes—Two Pairs of Genes

If we consider two pairs of genes with each pair carried on separate homologous chromosomes, the situation is somewhat different from that when one pair of alleles is involved. If we use pairs of genes A-a and B-b, nine different combinations of genes are possible in the individual: AABB, AABb, AAbb, AaBB, AaBb, Aabb, aaBB, aaBb, and aabb. Since genes (A) and (a) segregate independently from genes (B) and (b) in the gametes, we can use the law of probability which states that *the probability of two or more independent events occurring together is the product of each separate probability* to determine the probability of an individual of a certain genotype transmitting these genes to its offspring.

Suppose we have an individual of genotype AaBb, and we want to know what the probability would be that such an individual would transmit genes AB to an offspring. The probability of such an individual transmitting an (A) gene to an offspring is ½, and the probability of its transmitting a (B) gene to its offspring, is also $\frac{1}{2}$. Thus the probability of this individual transmitting the gene combination AB to an offspring is $\frac{1}{2} \times \frac{1}{2}$, or $\frac{1}{4}$. The probability of such an individual transmitting other combinations of genes to an offspring (such as Ab, aB, and ab) can also be calculated in the same manner. The probability of an AaBb individual transmitting any one of the three combinations of genes to an offspring is also $\frac{1}{4}$.

Segregation of Genes in the Gametes—Four Pairs of Genes

This same law of probability may also be used to calculate the probability that certain combinations of many pairs of genes may be transmitted to an offspring, providing each separate pair of genes is carried on separate pairs of homologous chromosomes and no new mutations occur. For example, the probability that an individual of genotype AaBbCcDd will transmit certain combinations of genes to an offspring is as follows:

P of transmitting ABCD is $\frac{1}{2} \times \frac{1}{2} \times \frac{1}{2} \times \frac{1}{2}$ or $\frac{1}{16}$

P of transmitting abcd is $\frac{1}{2} \times \frac{1}{2} \times \frac{1}{2} \times \frac{1}{2}$ or $\frac{1}{16}$

The same procedure is followed for calculating the probability that such an individual will transmit other combinations of genes to its offspring through the gametes.

Recombination of Genes in the Zygote—One Pair of Genes

The union of the sperm and the egg at fertilization restores the pairs of chromosomes and the pairs of genes carried on these chromosomes in the offspring, with one chromosome of each pair (as well as one gene of each pair) coming from each parent. We have previously shown that the paired genes in the potential parent segregate by chance into the gametes. The same law of chance also determines how these genes recombine in the offspring.

The recombination of genes in the offspring if both parents are of genotype Aa would have the following probabilities:

P of offspring carrying AA is $\frac{1}{2} \times \frac{1}{2}$ or $\frac{1}{4}$.

P of offspring carrying Aa is $2 (\frac{1}{2} \times \frac{1}{2})$ or $\frac{2}{4}$.

We multiply by 2 because Aa and aA are genetically identical.

P of offspring carrying aa is $\frac{1}{2} \times \frac{1}{2}$ or $\frac{1}{4}$.

Thus the recombination of genes in the zygote also follows the law of probability stated earlier.

Recombination of Genes in the Zygote—Two Pairs of Genes

Two or more pairs of genes carried in the gametes recombine in the zygote according to the law of chance mentioned previously, providing each pair of genes is carried on a different pair of homologous chromosomes and thus assort independently. If two pairs of genes are carried on the same pair of homologous chromosomes (known as linkage of genes) they are transmitted together in the gametes and do not assort independently except when crossing over occurs and genes on the two homologous chromosomes are exchanged during meiosis.

To illustrate the recombination of two pairs of genes in the zygote when each pair is carried on a different pair of homologous chromosomes, let us use the example where both parents are double heterozygotes, or AaBb. What is the probability that these two parents will have an offspring that is of genotype AABB? Taking each pair of genes separately, or one at a time, the probability of an AA offspring is ¼. Likewise, the probability of a BB offspring is ¼. Thus the probability of AA combining with BB in the offspring from such parents is ¼ × ¼ or ¹⁄₁₆. Using a similar procedure we can calculate the probability of such parents producing an offspring of any one of the other eight possible genotypes for these two pairs of genes. The probability of AaBb parents producing an AaBb offspring is ²⁄₄ × ²⁄₄ or ⁴⁄₁₆, and the probability of their producing an AaBB offspring is ²⁄₄ × ¼ or ²⁄₁₆.

The same procedure may be used to calculate the probability of parents of a known genotype producing a particular genotype in their offspring when more than two pairs of genes are involved, providing each pair of genes is carried on a separate pair of homologous chromosomes. For example, the probability of two parents of genotypes AaBbCcDd producing an AABBCCDD offspring is ¼ × ¼ × ¼ × ¼ or ¹⁄₂₅₆. The probability of other genotypes occurring in the offspring may be calculated by the same procedure.

PHENOTYPIC EXPRESSION OF GENES

Pairs of genes in the parent's body cells will segregate into half pairs in the sex cells and recombine in the offspring in the manner just described if the different pairs of genes are carried on separate pairs of homologous chromosomes in body cells. They segregate and recombine in this way regardless of how they might express themselves phenotypically (as seen or measured) in several different ways, and this has to be determined by experiments and observations. Much is now known about the phenotypic expression of genes.

Dominance and Recessiveness

A gene is dominant when it covers up or hides the phenotypic expression of another gene paired with it in the body cells. The gene whose phenotypic expression is hidden is called a recessive.

To illustrate this type of phenotypic expression of genes let us use the gene (B) for black coat color in horses which is dominant to gene (b) for the chestnut color. With these two genes (alleles), three genotypes and two phenotypes are possible as follows:

BB phenotype is black; genotype is homozygous dominant.

Bb phenotype is black; genotype is heterozygous dominant.

bb phenotype is chestnut; genotype is homozygous recessive.

Thus the gene for black (B) masks the phenotypic expression of gene (b) for chestnut in the heterozygous individual. When no dominant black gene (B) is present in the genotype, as in the chestnut (bb), the individual is able to express the recessive phenotype.

Several important genetic facts may now be stated. (1) A homozygous black (BB) parent always transmits a (B) gene to each offspring and will produce all black and no chestnut offspring regardless of whether the other parent is black or chestnut. (2) The heterozygous black (Bb) individual gives half of its offspring gene (B) and half gene (b), so it does not breed true. (3) The chestnut (bb) parent gives only the chestnut (b) gene to its offspring. If both parents are chestnut (bb), and if a mutation of (b) to (B) does not occur, all offspring will be chestnut. If one parent is black (BB or Bb), some or all of the offspring will be black. (4) Both black parents of a chestnut (bb) offspring would be of genotype (Bb) because the foal had to receive the chestnut gene (b) from both parents. What we have said about the dominant black gene (B) and the recessive chestnut gene (b) holds true for all other dominant and recessive genes in the individual.

Sometimes the dominant gene only partially covers up the phenotypic expression of its recessive mate. Such a dominant gene is said to be only partially dominant. In such cases one can tell the difference between the homozygous individuals from observation or certain tests. For example, red Shorthorn cattle are of genotype RR, roans are of genotype RW, and whites are of genotype WW. If, on the other hand, dominance were complete, one could not tell the difference between the homozygous dominant and the heterozygous dominant individuals by observation.

Overdominance

This type of phenotypic expression of genes means that the heterozygous individual is superior to either homozygote. With two genes (A and a) we can have three genotypes such as AA, Aa, and aa. In overdominance the Aa individual would be superior to either the AA or the aa genotypes. The individual does not breed true, however, but it can be produced almost 100% of the time by mating AA and aa parents. The overdominant action of genes seems to be important for traits related to physical fitness or vigor.

Epistasis

This may be defined as a type of phenotypic expression of genes in which one pair of genes affects the phenotypic expression of another pair of genes usually located on another pair of chromosomes. Two or more pairs of genes may be involved, but for illustrative purposes we will use only two pairs.

An example of epistasis is found in the dominant white coat color of horses. The dominant white gene (W) not only covers up the expression of its allele, the (w) gene that allows color when the genotype is ww, but it also hides or covers up the expression of the black (B) and the brown (b) genes as well as all other color genes. An individual of genotype WwBB would be white, whereas one of genotype wwBB would be black. This kind of gene action probably affects many traits in humans as well as other animals.

Additive Gene Action

In this type of phenotypic expression of genes there is no dominance, recessiveness, overdominance, or epistasis. Certain genes contribute something to the phenotype; others do not. The effects of different pairs of genes simply add to each other to give a more extreme phenotype. Many pairs of genes may affect the phenotype when additive gene action is involved, but we will again use only two different pairs of genes and assume that they are carried on two different pairs of homologous chromosomes. To illustrate this kind of gene action we will use a hypothetical example of speed in race horses. This trait seems to be affected by additive gene action because it is 35%–40% heritable, but more than the two pairs of genes we are using in this example may be involved. To illustrate additive gene action we will assume that genes (A) and (B) each contribute to greater speed, whereas genes (a) and (b) do not. The following genotypes and phenotypes would illustrate additive gene action:

aabb	poor racing ability
Aabb	less than average racing ability
AAbb or AaBb	average racing ability
AABb or aABB	above average racing ability
AABB	very good racing ability

Note that each time an (A) or (B) gene is added to the genotype, it adds to the faster racing ability of that individual. Thus the phenotypic effects add to each other.

Many traits in animals are determined by additive gene action and one can determine which trait by how highly heritable it is, with the higher the heritability the more variation that is due to additive gene action. Traits affected only by additive gene action do not express hybrid vigor nor are they affected adversely by inbreeding. Nonadditive gene action, which included dominance-recessiveness, overdominance, and epistasis, is indicated when the trait is very lowly heritable, expresses hybrid vigor when nonrelated parents are mated, and shows adverse effects when inbreeding is practiced. Since many traits in animals are affected by several pairs of genes, it is possible for some traits to be affected mostly by additive gene action, or mostly by nonadditive gene action, or by both.

Other Types of Phenotypic Expression of Genes

The mode of inheritance for a trait is changed somewhat from normal when the genes involved are carried on the sex chromosomes or when different sexes are involved. We will now present a few examples of these because some defects are affected by this type of inheritance, i.e., they are sex-linked.

As stated previously, each individual mammal carries one pair of chromosomes called the sex chromosomes, with one member of the pair being designated as the X and the other as the Y. The X chromosome in mammals is much longer than the Y and therefore must carry more genes. This is illustrated in Figure 1.3.

A sex-linked recessive trait is one in which the genes for the trait are carried on the portion of the X chromosome that has no counterpart (no homologous portion) in the Y. In the female mammal where two X chromosomes are present, the sex-linked recessive trait is inherited in exactly the same manner as other traits determined by a pair of recessive genes carried on the autosomes. These sex-linked genes are not paired in the male because he possesses only one X chromosome and the Y does not carry this gene. Therefore, in the male a sex-linked recessive trait needs only one recessive gene to express itself phenotypically and this recessive gene is always transmitted to the male mammal from its mother. This is true because each male mammal receives an X chromosome from its mother and a Y chromosome from its father. Female mammals, however, receive an X chromosome from both the father and mother. Sex-linked dominant traits can be transmitted from the sire to his daughters because he transmits an X chromosome to them, but he cannot transmit such a gene to his sons because he transmits only a Y chromosome to them. A mother could transmit a sex-linked dominant gene to either a son or daughter because she transmits an X chromosome to each of them and a gene of this kind is carried on the X chromosome.

A few genes may be carried on the nonhomologous portion of the Y chromosome (Fig. 1.3). Research workers do not all agree on what traits are determined in this manner, but apparently traits that might be carried on the nonhomologous portion of the Y are of little or no economic importance. Such traits would always be transmitted from a sire to his sons in subsequent generations. The inheritance due to genes on the nonhomologous portion of the Y chromosome is known a *holandric inheritance.*

Hologynic inheritance is a type of inheritance in which the mother always transmits the trait to her daughters and not to her sons. The theory used to explain this kind of inheritance is that the mother transmits two X chromosomes to her daughters, with none coming from the father.

The phenotypic expression of genes carried on the autosomes may be affected by the sex of the individual. In such cases, the trait is dominant in the male and recessive in the female, or one gene is necessary for the appearance of the trait in males and two in females. Baldness in humans and the presence of scurs (rudimentary horns) in English breeds of cattle are examples of this kind of inheritance.

Still another type of inheritance involving the sex of the individual is called sex-limited inheritance. Traits of this kind are limited to one sex, as a general rule. For example, only hens lay eggs and only cows give milk. The males of these species carry genes for these traits, but the genes cannot express themselves phenotypically in the males, perhaps because of the action and interaction of genes and sex hormones.

Other Variations in the Phenotypic Expression of Genes

It is possible for one gene to affect two or more traits in the individual. This is called *pleitrophy* and an example would be the situation in which some blue-eyed white cats are deaf. Coat color and other genetic defects have been described in many other species besides the cat.

Genes may express themselves at almost any time during the life of the individual. The mule-foot condition in swine is inherited and the gene expresses itself early in embryonic life when the hooves are being formed. Other traits may not appear in animals until much later in life. For example, baldness in humans is inherited but men are not usually bald until they are twenty or more years of age.

An individual may carry a gene for a certain trait but the trait may never be expressed. This is called a lack of *penetrance* of a gene and this makes it more difficult to eliminate such a gene from a group of animals. Also genes vary widely in their expression, as for example, dwarf calves vary from those that are definite dwarfs at birth to those that appear almost normal in size even when they reach maturity. *Varied expressivity* of genes also makes it more difficult to be certain of the genotype of the individual and increases the difficulty of eliminating a gene from a population.

The treatment of humans with certain drugs has shown that individuals differ genetically in their ability to inactivate some drugs in the body. An example is isoniazid, which is a drug used for the treatment of tuberculosis in humans. Some individuals inactivate this drug rather quickly in the body, and they possess homozygous dominant genes for inactivation. Other individuals are slow inactivators and they are homozygous recessive. Heterozygous dominant individuals are intermediate between the two other genotypes in the rapidity of inactivity of this drug. In some slow inactivators, toxic symptoms appear as polyneuritis due to the continued presence of the drug in the body. About 50% of the people in the United States and Europe are slow inactivators. No doubt mammals other than humans may be susceptible to certain drugs administered for the treatment of illnesses and, with prolonged use, some toxic symptoms may appear.

CONTROLLING AND ELIMINATING RECESSIVE GENES IN A POPULATION

Most genetic defects in animals are either recessive or partially dominant in their phenotypic expression. The defects due to a dominant gene probably would be eliminated because the individuals possessing such a defect would be less likely to survive than the normal individuals. Therefore, in most instances animal breeders are confronted with the elimination of a recessive gene from their herd, kennel, or cattery and this is much harder to do than to eliminate a dominant or partially dominant gene. Carriers of a dominant or partially dominant gene can be identified by eye appraisal and eliminated. Carriers (heterozygotes) of a completely recessive gene are not distinguishable from those of the homozygous dominant phenotype. Therefore, special methods are necessary to identify and eliminate a recessive gene from herds, kennels, etc.

To eliminate a recessive gene, all the homozygous recessive individuals must be culled as well as their parents, because their parents are also carriers of that recessive gene. All other carriers of the recessive gene must be identified and culled. This requires a breeding test, unless other tests are available, to determine if the individual of the dominant phenotype is homozygous or heterozygous. In animals that give birth to 1 young (primiparous), it is almost impossible to progeny test females because it may take many years and many progeny for the test to be completed. In litter-bearing animals (multiparous), such a test is possible in females as well as males.

The most practical test for identifying a dominant carrier of a recessive gene, if homozygous recessive individuals for this trait survive and are fertile, is to mate the animals to be tested to at least 5 homozygous recessive individuals or at least produce 5 offspring from a recessive individual. If a recessive offspring is produced, it is proof that the animal being tested is heterozygous dominant. Five offspring of the dominant phenotype from such matings without a recessive offspring produced are proof that the animal being tested is homozygous dominant at the 95% confidence level of probability. Seven such matings without a homozygous recessive offspring being produced are proof that the animal tested is homozygous dominant at the 99% level of probability.

Sometimes the homozygous recessive individuals die early in life or are infertile and cannot be used for testing purposes. In such a case the test matings may be made with the animal of the dominant phenotype (animal being tested) mated with known dominant carriers of the recessive gene. An individual is a known carrier of a recessive gene if it is of the dominant phenotype but has produced 1 offspring that is recessive or has had 1 parent that is recessive. Again, 1 recessive offspring from such a mating proves the individual being tested heterozygous dominant, whereas 11 such matings without a homozygous recessive offspring being produced are proof that the tested individual is homozygous dominant at the 95% level of probability. Sixteen dominant and no recessive offspring from such matings prove the individual being tested homozygous dominant at the 99% level of probability.

In litter-bearing animals, it is possible to mate the individual to be tested to 1 female that is homozygous recessive to prove its genotype. One recessive offspring from such a mating proves the animal being tested heterozygous dominant. Five offspring of the dominant phenotype without a recessive offspring produced prove the animal being tested homozygous dominant at the 95% level of probability, whereas 7 dominant and no recessive offspring prove the animal being tested homozygous dominant at the 99% probability level. If heterozygous individuals are used for testing in multiparous animals, 11 offspring of the dominant phenotype or 16 offspring of the dominant phenotype without a recessive offspring prove the animal being tested homozygous dominant at the 95% or 99% level of probability, respectively.

Another method of testing an individual of the dominant phenotype to determine if it is homozygous or heterozygous dominant is to mate it to its own progeny. In primiparous animals this is practical only for males, whereas in multiparous animals both males and females can be progeny tested for a recessive gene in this manner. The advantage of this testing method is that it is possible to test for any recessive gene the individual might be carrying and not for just a specific one. A disadvantage is that the offspring are at least 25% inbred and may lack vigor or some of them may even show a genetic defect that hinders their performance. A single recessive offspring produced from such a mating proves the animal being tested a carrier of a recessive gene. In primiparous animals, 23 offspring from 23 different unselected daughters with no recessive offspring produced prove the male being tested homozygous dominant at the 95% level of probability, whereas 35 progeny from 35 different unselected daughters and no recessive offspring produced prove the male being tested homozygous dominant for all recessive defective genes at the 99% level of probability. In multiparous animals a parent mated to 5 of its unselected offspring with at least 11 progeny produced from each mating with no recessive offspring produced is proof at the 95% level of probability that the parent is homozygous dominant, or free from recessive defects. A parent mated to 7 unselected offspring with 16 progeny produced per mating and none of which are homozygous recessive proves the individual being tested free from recessive defects at the 99% level of probability.

QUANTITATIVE INHERITANCE

The previous discussion dealt with some basic principles of genetics in which only one or two pairs of genes were involved and there was a sharp distinction between phenotypes. This is known as *qualitative inheritance.* Traits such as speed, mature height, rate and efficiency of gain, milk production, and many others are usually determined by many pairs of genes, and the phenotypes are not sharply distinct from one another, and environment as well as heredity affects these traits. This is called *quantitative inheritance.* Most of the traits (defects) discussed here will deal with qualitative inheritance, so we will not elaborate on methods of improving livestock animals through attention to quantitative methods. Quantitative inheritance is involved sometimes, however, in resistance to disease or to deficiencies in the diet. Quantitative inheritance may also be important for breeds having height limitations, etc.

Inbreeding

Inbreeding is one of the tools available to the breeder for the improvement of his animals. It may be defined as the production of offspring by parents more closely related to each other than the average of the population. Some breeders have erroneously considered close inbreeding (such as brother-sister, father-daughter) as inbreeding and less intense (grandfather-granddaughter) as linebreeding. Both are inbreeding.

Inbreeding is usually practiced for one or more reasons. In the initial stages of the development of a breed, inbreeding is necessary because the small nucleus of animals forming the breed is closed to outside blood and this limits the number of breeding stock available. These top breeding animals are usually related.

Inbreeding was practiced in the development of almost every breed of livestock. It was even used in the early history of the human race. Moses was inbred because the same ancestor, Terah, appeared in his pedigree at least twelve times. Terah was so far back in Moses's pedigree, however, that the amount of inbreeding was small, ranging between 5% and 6%.

Many breeders of purebred companion animals routinely practice inbreeding. Perhaps one of the reasons for this is that some individual has an outstanding show record and there is tendency to breed as many females as possible to such a male. In later generations an attempt is often made to concentrate the inheritance of this ancestor by linebreeding.

WHAT INBREEDING DOES GENETICALLY. Inbreeding tends to make animals more homozygous for the genes they carry. In other words, the genes of each pair they carry in their body cells are more likely to be alike. The proportional increase in the pairs of homozygous genes in the inbred offspring increases with the intensity or amount of inbreeding. The more closely the parents are related, the more intense the inbreeding or the increase in homozygosity. Homozygosity increases with more intense inbreeding regardless of how genes express themselves phenotypically. Thus dominant, recessive, partially dominant, overdominant, and additive genes are made more homozygous. The increase in homozygosity is estimated from the inbreeding coefficient. For example, if an animal is inbred by 25%, or the equivalent of being produced from the mating of a full brother with a full sister, the percentage of genes made homozygous is increased by 25% over those that were homozygous before inbreeding was practiced. If an animal is inbred by 12.5%, or the equivalent of a half-brother × half-sister mating, the increase in the percentage of homozygous genes over what was present in the population before inbreeding was practiced is 12.5%. Thus higher inbreeding makes more pairs of genes homozygous. The amount of inbreeding to expect from some different kinds of mating is given in Table 1.2.

Table 1.2. Percentage of inbreeding in offspring produced by different kinds of matings when parents are not inbred.

Type of Mating	% of Inbreeding in Offspring
Parent × offspring	25.00
Full brother × full sister	25.00
Half-brother × half-sister	12.50
First cousins	6.25
Second cousins	1.56
Third cousins	0.39
Nephew × aunt or niece × uncle	12.50
Grandparent × grandchild	12.50
Double first cousins	12.50

Increased homozygosity increases the probability that all offspring will receive the same inheritance from their inbred parent. We can illustrate this by the following example using four different pairs of genes, each pair of which is inherited independently of the others:

Animal 1 . . . . . AABBCCDD (homozygous for four pairs of genes).

Animal 2 . . . . . AaBbCcDd (heterozygous for four pairs of genes).

Animal 1 will transmit the same genes, ABCD, to each of its offspring. Animal 2 will transmit one of 16 different combinations of genes to each offspring. Obviously, the majority of offspring from animal 1 would resemble each other and that parent much more than would the offspring of animal 2. The unusual resemblance of offspring to each other or to their parent is called prepotency.

WHAT TO EXPECT FROM INBREEDING. Inbreeding will cause inherited recessive traits to appear if the parental stock carry the recessive genes. Recessive traits are usually undesirable. If recessive genes are not present in the original breeding stock, increased inbreeding cannot uncover such genes or cause them to appear. Inbreeding does not create new recessive genes, it just allows them to express themselves. Noninbred individuals probably already carry one or more of several recessive detrimental genes covered up by dominant genes that may not appear unless inbreeding is practiced.

Increased inbreeding causes a reduction in fertility in some instances. Reduced fertility is due to a poorer conception rate or to a higher fetal death loss, probably because of the pairing of detrimental recessive or partially dominant genes in the new individual.

Increased inbreeding causes a decline in those traits related to physical fitness. The most dramatic effect here is the lowered viability observed in inbred animals. The death rate shortly after birth is higher in inbred than in noninbred individuals. Inbred individuals may also lack somewhat in size, although this is not always true.

Inbred individuals when mated to nonrelated animals will tend to breed better than they look. Outbred individuals, on the other hand, tend to look better than they breed. Breeders seldom, if ever, recognize this and pay no more for inbred or linebred individuals than for noninbred stock. In fact, they often will pay less because individuals that are inbred may not be so desirable in size, health, type, and performance.

THE PURPOSE OF INBREEDING. One reason for inbreeding in certain species is to produce lines for crossing. This is well illustrated by the procedures followed in the production of hybrid seed corn. Corn is naturally an open-pollinated plant with the tassels of each plant being fertilized by pollen from other plants in the same field. A cornstalk possesses both male and female parts. Thus the use of pollen from a corn plant to fertilize the same corn plant results in self-fertilization. Self-fertilization in the first cross results in a 50% increase in the pairs of homozygous genes in the inbred individual. This is another way of saying that inbreeding is increased by 50%. After several generations of inbreeding, the line approaches 100% inbreeding with almost all pairs of genes homozygous. With the increased inbreeding (homozygosity), some inbred lines fail to maintain themselves because of severe decreased vigor or the appearance of lethal (death causing) recessive defects. Inbred lines decrease somewhat in vigor but some survive. When homozygosity approaches 100%, the various surviving lines are crossed to find those that cross the best as shown by the performance of their linecross offspring. Those that cross the best are kept as pure lines and crossed from time to time to produce linecross seed which is sold to farmers to plant for the commercial production of corn. Since the inbred lines are genetically pure, if they cross well one time they should continue to cross well at later times. The inbred lines must be kept pure; however, certain methods may be used to improve each line when that becomes necessary.

Very few animal breeders, and especially not breeders of companion animals, inbreed with the objective of producing two or more inbred lines for crossing. They usually inbreed to produce superior individuals. Often superior individuals are produced through inbreeding, but on the average, inbreds (for certain traits) are likely to show a decline as inbreeding increases. Then, too, some recessive traits appear that are quite detrimental and undesirable. Therefore, it is very difficult, if not impossible, to develop inbred lines of animals (especially economic species) that will perform as well as those that are not inbred. The breeder should always keep this in mind when following an inbreeding program.

To most livestock breeders any amount of inbreeding gives undesirable results. Perhaps this is because few know how to calculate the amount of inbreeding. Nevertheless, the more intense the inbreeding, the more likely the individuals are to lack vigor and the more likely recessive traits will appear if they were present in the original parental stock.

Linebreeding

Linebreeding is a form of inbreeding in which an attempt is made to keep the relationship of individuals in the herd or kennel, etc., as high as possible to some outstanding ancestor in the pedigree. The ancestor is usually a male rather than a female because he has so many more descendants, as a general rule, and this allows a greater opportunity to prove his merit by means of a progeny test.

Pedigree 1 is given to illustrate systematic linebreeding (Fig. 1.8). Letters are used in place of names to make the handling of the pedigree simpler. Only one ancestor in this pedigree is responsible for the relationship between the sire and dam of individual X. This ancestor is individual F. We have purposely placed him in the pedigree as the only great-grandsire of individual X. The arrow diagram shows that individual X traces by four separate lines to ancestor F. This illustrates why it is called linebreeding. By looking at pedigree 1, it can be seen that individual X received approximately 50% of his inheritance from ancestor F, his great-grandfather. A correction for the inbreeding of individual X would lower this figure to about 47%. Thus the relationship between individual X and his ancestor F is approximately as great as it usually is between a sire and his offspring (50%). If linebreeding had not been practiced, the relationship between X and F would have been only 12.5% or they would have approximately this propor-

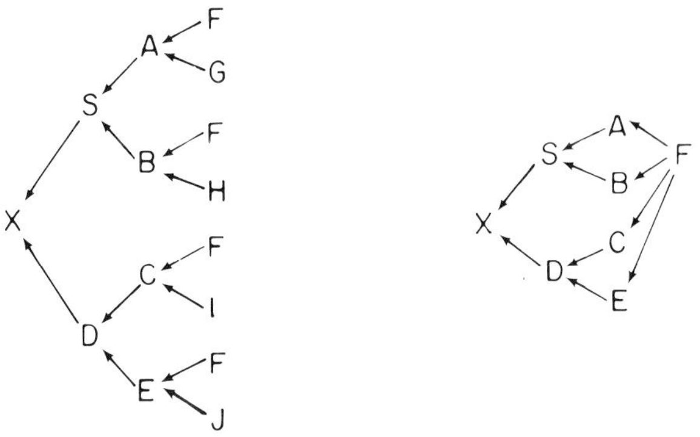

PEDIGREE   ARROW DIAGRAM

Fig. 1.8. *This pedigree and arrow diagram illustrate a definite system of linebreeding where an attempt has been made to concentrate the blood of individual F in the pedigree. Individual X is inbred about 12.5% and the relationship between X and F is slightly less than 50%.*

tion of their inheritance in common. Table 1.3 gives the relationship between an individual and his various ancestors.

Several generations of linebreeding to some ancestor will eventually require linebreeding through some of his descendants, but the attempt is still made to concentrate the inheritance of the desired individual.

COMPARISON OF ORDINARY INBREEDING AND LINEBREEDING. As previously stated, linebreeding is inbreeding but not all inbreeding is linebreeding. In

Table 1.3. Probable percentage of genes (relationship) that an individual has in common with his ancestors

Kind of Ancestor	% of Blood	% of Relationship
No Inbreeding Involved:		
A parent	50.00	
A grandparent	25.00	
A great-grandparent	12.50	
A great-great-grandparent	6.25	
Inbreeding Involved:		
Both a parent and a grandparent*	75.00	67.08
A double grandparent	50.00	47.14
A double great-grandparent†	25.00	24.62
A triple great-grandparent	37.50	36.38
A quadruple great-grandparent	50.00	47.14

* Individual resulting from the mating of a sire to his own daughter or a dam to her own son.

† The same individual is a grandparent of both the sire and dam. If a double great-grandparent only in the sire's or in the dam's pedigree, the relationship would not have to be corrected for inbreeding and would be 25.00%.

pedigree 1 where linebreeding was illustrated, individual X was inbred by
about 12.5%. Most people would look at the pedigree and say that X was
intensely inbred. This really is not true because only one individual was
responsible for the inbreeding of X and this ancestor was found back in the
third generation.

Inbreeding may be defined as the production of offspring from parents
more closely related to each other than to the average of the population.
Linebreeding is actually a special form of inbreeding. Ordinary inbreeding
is the mating of relatives, but there is no attempt to keep the relationship to
any one particular ancestor high in the pedigree. In fact, several ancestors
may be responsible for the inbreeding. Let us change the letters in pedigree 1
to form pedigree 2 to illustrate this point (Fig. 1.9). The arrow diagram of
pedigree 2 shows that four different ancestors are responsible for the inbreeding of X. The inbreeding of X is still 12.5% as in pedigree 1, but the
relationship of ancestor F to X is less than 12.5%. Thus in this pedigree
there has been inbreeding without an attempt to concentrate the blood of
any one particular ancestor. This is a rather complex pedigree, but it illustrates the difference between ordinary inbreeding and linebreeding.
These illustrations are extreme and in some pedigrees it is difficult to
distinguish between ordinary inbreeding and linebreeding.

WHEN TO LINEBREED. This is an important point. Linebreeding should be used
only in the production of purebreds and one should never linebreed just to
be linebreeding. Such a program might be interesting but probably would be
of little value. In fact, linebreeding in such an instance might result in the
production of inferior animals.

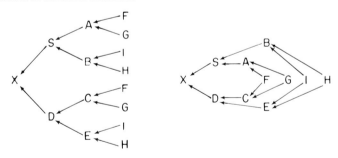

PEDIGREE   ARROW DIAGRAM

Fig. 1.9. *This pedigree and arrow diagram illustrate a form of
inbreeding that is not linebreeding because four different ancestors (F, G, I, and H) are responsible for the inbreeding and no
attempt has been made to concentrate the blood of any one
ancestor. Individual X is inbred about 12.5% and the
relationship between X and F is less than 12.5%.*

The use of linebreeding is indicated when some truly outstanding individual in the breed has been identified and proved superior by an adequate progeny test. If such an individual is still living and available for breeding purposes, it seems more desirable to use him as a sire since all his sons and daughters are related to him by 50%.

Linebreeding may be practiced when the outstanding individual is dead or not available for breeding purposes. A system of linebreeding illustrated in pedigree 1 should be followed when possible or various modifications of this system could be used. The main point is to concentrate the blood of the outstanding ancestor as much as possible. This requires a planned, systematic mating system. The system illustrated in pedigree 1 cannot be followed indefinitely and sooner or later linebreeding must be directed through some of his sons and daughters, usually his sons. This is illustrated in pedigree 3 (Fig. 1.10).

Linebreeding to a particularly outstanding sire may be practiced by a breeder who does not own the sire, cannot purchase him, or cannot obtain his services. If he can purchase or use one or more high quality sons and daughters of the admired ancestor, he can practice the linebreeding illustrated in pedigrees 1 and 3 and increase the relationship of offspring in the herd, kennel, etc., to the outstanding individual.

HOW TO USE LINEBREEDING. The following points are recommendations on how to use linebreeding:

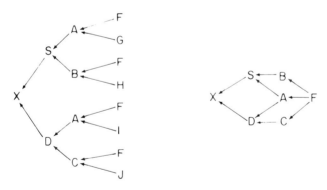

PEDIGREE   ARROW DIAGRAM

Fig. 1.10. *This pedigree and arrow diagram show a system of linebreeding to individual F through his son A. Individual X is inbred by 21.875% and the relationship between X and F is about 50%. Note that the inbreeding of individual X is higher in this system of linebreeding than it is in the system shown in pedigree 1. However, it requires just one son of individual F in this system whereas at least two are required in pedigree 1.*

1. Linebreed only when some outstanding individual has been identified by a satisfactory progeny test and not on just someone's opinion.
2. Be ready to cull rigorously in the linebred individuals.
3. Depart from linebreeding if some undesirable fault appears. Be on the lookout for such faults.
4. Do not breed too closely. The mating of a sire to his own daughters is as close breeding as possible and may be used to determine any recessive genetic defects the sire is carrying. Half-sister × half-brother matings similar to those in pedigree 1 are probably close enough in most cases. If one desires to make a father × daughter mating, one should be aware of possible consequences.
5. When superior linebred families are developed, crosses of two or more of them would improve the performance traits, such as vigor, etc., of the linecross offspring. If other linebred families are not available, outcross to some desired individual where greater vigor and performance are desired. However, keep the linebred family intact for seedstock production if it is superior. Just one outcross results in the offspring no longer being linebred. Certain traits might not be improved by the crossing of linebred families.

Outbreeding

This mating system may be defined as the production of offspring from unrelated parents or less related than the average within a breed. At least the parents are not related within the last four or five generations.

The genotypic and phenotypic effects (on certain traits) of outbreeding are exactly opposite to those of inbreeding and linebreeding. Outbreeding increases heterozygosity of the outbred individuals, it tends to cover up recessive or partially dominant genes, and it is usually accompanied by an improvement in traits related to physical fitness. It is the mating system most often followed by breeders of purebred animals who try to avoid inbreeding and linebreeding. In general, outbreeding tends to decrease breeding purity because more pairs of genes are made heterozygous. Thus an outbred individual is more likely to look better than it breeds, although there are some exceptions.

Crossbreeding

This system of mating is the production of offspring by mating individuals from two or more breeds. Crossbreeding is rarely used (intentionally) in companion animals. It gives the same results as outbreeding, although the genotypic and phenotypic effects are more extreme. Crossbreeding produces traits that show hybrid vigor and is used because of this in the commercial production of many plants and animals, especially poultry, swine, and cattle. Crossbreeding, as well as outbreeding, tends to cover up recessive genes in the offspring. However, it is possible for crossbred individuals to show a genetic defect that did not appear in either of the pure breeds used for making the cross. For example, let us assume that a combination of genes (A) and (B) as (A_B_) are responsible for the occurrence of a defect. If one parent were aaBB and the other AAbb, all offspring would be AaBb and would show a defect not seen in either parent.

PART II

Abnormalities
of the Dog

Section A:

DEFECTS WITH A PROBABLE GENETIC BASE

SUMMARY OF DEFECTS BY BREED

The following is a summary list of structural and functional defects found in the dog that have been reported or suggested to have a genetic base by the authors given in the reference sections following each defect.

Some of the defects are rarely observed. Many of the defects are found in many of the breeds; certain defects have been reported for only one breed. Limited data prevent definite conclusions as to whether some of these traits are inherited.

The numbers listed under the defects are coded for the breeds in which the condition is most common and/or at least has been reported. For additional information as to inheritance, see the text.

BLOOD AND IMMUNE SYSTEM

Canine cyclic neutropenia, 33
Congenital hemolytic anemia, 5, 8, 10
Congenital hereditary lymphoedema, 129
Fibrinogen deficiencies, 33, 114
Hemophilia (factor VII), 5, 10
Hemophilia (factor XI), 47, 109
Hemophilia (factor X), 107
Hemophilia A (factor VIII), 10, 31, 33, 43, 44, 48, 86, 90, 95, 97, 98, 100, 117, 118
Hemophilia B (factor IX), 18, 30, 43, 107, 114
Platelet function defects, 9, 39, 70, 93
Von Willebrand's disease, 37, 44, 65, 83, 93

CARDIOVASCULAR SYSTEM

Aortic stenosis, 24, 27, (41 & 42), 44, 66, 109
Atrial septal defect, 24
Patent ductus arteriosus, 33, 76, 77, 107
Persistent right aortic arch, 22, 44, 97

Pulmonic stenosis, 10, 27, 31, (41 & 42), 45, 65, 90, 115
Tetralogy of Fallot, 54
Ventricular septal defect, 100

SENSORY ORGANS

Ear
Deafness, 29, 33, 34, 35, 39, (41 & 42), 46, 77, 78, 79, 88, 93, 94, 98, 127

Eye
Cataracts, 2, 6, 10, 22, (41 & 42), 65, 69, 73, 77, 78, 79, 85, 86, 107
Central progressive retinal atrophy, 85, 86, 98, 109, 127
Collie eye anomaly, 33
Dermoid cyst of cornea, 9, 27, 34, 44, 66, 107, 114, 118, (119 & 120)
Distichia, 12, 22, 24, 27, 31, 32, 33, 34, 42, 44, 72, 76, 77, 78, 79, 80, 86, 98, 107, 109
Ectropion, 9, 19, 27, 46, 63, 95, 97, 107, 114

35

Entropion, 19, 24, 27, 28, 32, 51, 67, 71, 76, 77, 78, 79, 85, 86, 97, 107, 109, 114, 128

Glaucoma, 9, 10, 107

Hemeralopia, 5, 77

Everted membrana nictitans, 44, 46, 66, 74, 114, 118

Luxation of lens, 41, 42, 43, 44, 48, 86, 93, 94, 119, 120, 127

Microphthalmia, 126

Persistent pupillary membrane, 8

Progressive retinal atrophy, 4, 33, 64, 67, 77, 79, 85, 86, 89, 90, 97, 100, 107, 108, 128

Retinal dysplasia, 12, 86, 94

Superficial indolent ulcer of cornea, 24

Trichiasis, 27, 31, 34, 41, 42, 72, 77, 78, 79, 80, 98

BONES AND JOINTS

Achondroplasia, 128

Anury, 107

Brachyury, 10, 26, 107

Carpal subluxation, none given

Cartilaginous exostoses, 5, 125, 129

Cervical vertebral deformity, 9, 37, (41 & 42), 46, 69, 87, 97, 114

Craniomandibular osteopathy, 77, 79, 86, 93, 122

Cranioschisis (skull fissures), 107

Dwarfism, 5, 98

Epiphyseal dysplasia, 10, 77

Foramen magnum, 31, 102, 107

Hemivertebra, 22, 27, 43

Hip dysplasia, 128

Intertarsal and tarsometarsal subluxation, 33, 98

Intervertebral disc degeneration, 10, 34, 43, 59, 72, 77, 99, 107, 119, 120, 128

Legg-Calvé-Perthes disease, 61, 62, 65, 72, 77, 79, 80, 128 (small)

Osteogenesis imperfecta, 12, 67, 78

Otocephaly, none given

Overshot jaw, 34, 107

Panosteitis (enostosis), 44

Patellar luxation, 22, 26, 31, 43, 72, 76, 77, 98, 107, 125, 128 (small)

Polydactyly, 128

Polyostotic fibrous dysplasia, 37

Short spine (spina bifida), 10

Spondylitis deformans, 3, 24, 34, 43, 44, 107, 128

Undershot jaw, 22, 27, 72

Ununited anconeal process, 9, 19, 28, 34, 43, 44, 46, 47, 51, 58, 66, 73, 114, 118

Vertebral osteochondrosis, 39

NEUROMUSCULAR SYSTEM

Ataxia, 3, 22, 41, 43, 93

Brachycephalic, 31, 61, 62, 72

Cerebellar cortical and extrapyramidal nuclear abiotrophy, 55

Cerebellar hypoplasia, 3

Cerebrospinal demyelination, 77

Epilepsy, 10, 15, 33, 34, 44, 54, 74, 77, 107, 128

Familial amaurotic idiocy gangliosidosis, 10, 30, 77, 122

Globoid leukodystrophy, 30, 122

Hydrocephalus, 128

Lissencephaly, 59

Muscle fiber deficiency, 86

Neuronal ceroid-lipofuscinosis, none given

Scottie cramp, 93

Spinal dysraphism (syringomyelia), 118

Stockard's paralysis, 19, 46, 114, 129

Trembling, 3

DIGESTIVE SYSTEM

Cleft lip and palate, 129 (brachycephalic), 6, 10, 16, 22, 24, 27, 28, 29, 31, 33, 34, 44, 67, 72, 79, 99, 107

Esophageal achalasia, 22, 24, 41, 44, 48, 86, 87, 109, 129

Gingival hyperplasia, 24

Intestinal lymphangiectasia, 8

Liver disease, 12

ENDOCRINE AND METABOLIC SYSTEM

Diabetes mellitus, 34, 129

Glycogen storage disease, 129 (small)

Goiter, (41 & 42)

Pituitary dwarfism, 44

UROGENITAL SYSTEM

Cryptorchidism, 129

Cystinuria, 129

Familial renal disease, 67

Intersexuality, 129

Polycystic kidney disease, 129

Renal agenesis and dysgenesis, 10, 129

Renal cortical hypoplasia, 34, 44, 59, 67, 107

Uric acid excretion, 35

SKIN APPENDAGES AND CONNECTIVE TISSUE

Atopic dermatitis, 35, 42, 128
Black hair follicular dysplasia, 129
Blue dog syndrome, 34, 37, 46, 123
Cutaneous asthenia, 10, 61, 62, 109,
   119, 120, 129
Dermoid sinus, 87
Ectodermal defect, 77, 107, 123
Hairlessness, 77, 123

OTHER STRUCTURES

Calcinosis circumscripta (ca-gout), 24,
   29, 44, 46, 48, 51, 73, 86, 129
   (large)
Diaphragmatic hernia, 128, 129
Glossopharyngeal defect (bird tongue),
   none given
Inguinal hernia, 8, 9, 30, 72, 122, 128
Laryngeal-tracheal collapse, 128 (toy)
Umbilical hernia, 3, 8, 29, 33, 72, 73,
   107, 118, 128

DOG BREEDS

1. Affenpinscher
2. Afghan hound
3. Airedale terrier
4. Akita
5. Alaskan malamute
6. American Stafford-
   shire terrier
7. Australian terrier
8. Basenji
9. Basset hound
10. Beagle
11. Bearded collie
12. Bedlington terrier
13. Belgian Malinois
14. Belgian sheepdog
15. Belgian Tervuren
16. Bernese mountain
   dog
17. Bichon Frise
18. Black-and-tan
   coonhound
19. Bloodhound
20. Border terrier
21. Borzois
22. Boston terrier
23. Bouvier des Flandres
24. Boxer
25. Briard
26. Brussels griffon
27. Bulldog
28. Bullmastiff
29. Bull terrier
30. Cairn terrier
31. Chihuahua
32. Chow chow
33. Collie
34. Dachshund

35. Dalmatian
36. Dandie Dinmont
   terrier
37. Doberman pinscher
38. English toy spaniel
39. Foxhound (American)
40. Foxhound (English)
41. Fox terrier (smooth)
42. Fox terrier (wire)
43. French bulldog
44. German shepherd
   dog
45. Giant schnauzer
46. Great Dane
47. Great Pyrenees
48. Greyhounds
49. Harrier
50. Irish terrier
51. Irish wolfhound
52. Italian greyhound
53. Japanese spaniel
54. Keeshond
55. Kerry blue terrier
56. Komondorok
57. Kuvaszok
58. Lakeland terrier
59. Lhasa Apso
60. Maltese
61. Manchester terrier
   (standard)
62. Manchester terrier
   (toy)
63. Mastiff
64. Miniature pinscher
65. Miniature schnauzer
66. Newfoundland
67. Norwegian elkhound

68. Norwich terrier
69. Old English sheep-
   dog
70. Otter hound
71. Papillon
72. Pekingese
73. Pointer
74. Pointer (German
   shorthaired)
75. Pointer (German
   wirehaired)
76. Pomeranian
77. Poodle (miniature)
78. Poodle (standard)
79. Poodle (toy)
80. Pug
81. Pulik
82. Retriever (Chesa-
   peake Bay)
83. Retriever (curly
   coated)
84. Retriever (flat
   coated)
85. Retriever (golden)
86. Retriever (Labra-
   dor)
87. Rhodesian Ridge-
   back
88. Rottweiler
89. Saluki
90. Samoyed
91. Schipperke
92. Scottish deerhound
93. Scottish terrier
94. Sealyham terrier
95. Setter (English)
96. Setter (Gordon)

97. Setter (Irish)
98. Shetland sheepdog
99. Shih Tzu
100. Siberian huskie
101. Silky terrier
102. Skye terrier
103. Soft-coated Wheaton terrier
104. Spaniel (American water)
105. Spaniel (Brittany)
106. Spaniel (Clumber)
107. Spaniel (cocker)
108. Spaniel (English cocker)
109. Spaniel (English springer)
110. Spaniel (field)
111. Spaniel (Irish water)
112. Spaniel (Sussex)
113. Spaniel (Welsh springer)
114. Saint Bernard
115. Standard schnauzer
116. Tibetan terrier
117. Vizsla
118. Weimaraner
119. Welsh corgi (Cardigan)
120. Welsh corgi (Pembroke)
121. Welsh terrier
122. West Highland white terrier
123. Whippet
124. Wirehaired pointing griffon
125. Yorkshire terrier
   (not AKC breeds)
126. Australian shepherd
127. Border collie
128. Many breeds
129. Crossbreeds

CHAPTER 2

Hemopoietic and Lymphatic Systems

HEMORRHAGIC (COAGULATION) DEFECTS

The precise mechanism by which blood clots is not well known. Over thirty different substances have been suggested to be involved. Most authors agree that there are three essential steps in blood coagulation. The first essential step is the formation of the prothrombin activator. This step is complex. This first step may be initiated in one of two ways. One way, the extrinsic mechanism, initially involves an extract (thromboplastin) from the damaged tissue. The other way, the intrinsic mechanism, involves an important substance released from the platelets (platelet factor III). Both mechanisms involve a series of special protein factors (extrinsic: factors VII, V, and X; intrinsic: factors VII, IX, XI, XII, V, and X) found in blood plasma. For normal clotting these factors must be present in proper sequence for the stepwise, progressive formation of the prothrombin activator. If all clotting factors are present (the protein; plus calcium, thromboplastin, platelet factor III, etc.), the end result is the production of the extrinsic prothrombin activator or the intrinsic prothrombin activator or both, depending on which pathway was followed. The second essential step is that the prothrombin activator catalyzes the conversion of prothrombin into thrombin. The third step is that thrombin acts as an enzyme to convert fibrinogen into fibrin threads that trap the red blood cells and plasma to form the clot.

Hemophilia A (Factor VIII Deficiency)

The most common form of hemophilia found in the dog is hemophilia A, which is the result of a deficiency of factor VIII. This condition occurs in many breeds including the Irish setter, English setter,

Labrador, German shepherd, beagle, Weimaraner, Chihuahua, collie, vizsla, Siberian husky, greyhound, Samoyed, Shetland sheepdog, French bulldog, and some crossbreeds. Hemophilia A may be observed in pups at birth, expressed as persistent bleeding from the umbilical cord, which may require ligation to prevent fatal hemorrhage. Normally the hemophilic condition is first observed when the puppies are 6 weeks to 3 months of age. Affected dogs often develop unilateral or bilateral (one or both sides) joint enlargement, due to periarticular (around the joint) hemorrhage and hemarthrosis (hemorrhage into a joint). Hemarthrosis is painful and causes lameness. It is more severe in larger dogs, since the extra weight on the joints predisposes them to spontaneous hemarthrosis. Limbs may or may not be swollen. Bleeding may occur in the gastrointestinal tract or other tissues. Gastrointestinal bleeding could result in a discoloration of the stool. Subsequent development of lumps, which are actually hematomata (accumulation of blood), occurs throughout the body. Anorexia (loss of appetite) is a common characteristic of hemophilic dogs.

PATHOPHYSIOLOGY. Canine hemophilia A results from a deficiency of factor VIII. Therefore, the dogs have a markedly defective intrinsic clotting mechanism. Factor VIII is required as a cofactor, along with other factors, in the presence of platelet factor 3 and calcium to activate factor X and form the intrinsic prothrombin activator. Studies in dogs show that in hemophilia the primary platelet plug contains more vascular channels than normal and there is less fibrin in contact with collagen at the edge of the wound. The plugs are easily dislodged with subsequent rebleeding, and secondary plugs form with difficulty, there being little fibrin deposited.

Affected animals have markedly defective intrinsic clotting (long whole blood clotting, plasma recalcification, and partial thromboplastin times; very short prothrombin consumption or plasma clotting times). The extrinsic clotting (prothrombin and Russell's viper venom times) and platelet function are normal. It has been found that the factor VIII level in a dog with severe bleeding is less than 1% of that in the normal dog, 1%–5% in moderately affected animals, and 5%–20% in those with mild bleeding problems. The factor VIII level in carriers is usually about 40%–60% of normal. Hemophiliac and carrier bitches have normal to increased levels of factor VIII–related antigen, in contrast to their decreased factor VIII activities.

INHERITANCE AND RECOMMENDATION. Hemophilia A is inherited as a sex-linked recessive, with the gene for the defect carried on the nonhomologous portion of the X chromosome. Because the gene is located on the

X chromosome, one would most frequently observe the hemophilic condition in the male, but one should be aware that with certain matings it will also appear in the female.

Dogs showing hemophilia should not be used for breeding. Males present no problem since males that do not show the hemophilic trait are normal and do not transmit hemophilia to their offspring. Males having the disease would transmit it to their daughters. Since the gene is carried on the X chromosome, there are no carrier males. The female, on the other hand, could appear normal but be a carrier for hemophilia. Hemophilic females that have the disease would be obvious. A breeding test could be conducted to prove the bitch normal or a carrier. A bitch could be bred to an affected or nonaffected male. At least five male pups free from hemophilia would be required to establish a 95% degree of confidence that the female in question was not a carrier. Blood tests could also be run on the bitches to detect the carriers.

Hemophilia B (Factor IX Deficiency)

Hemophilia B is a factor IX deficiency that has been reported in cairn terriers, Saint Bernards, French bulldogs, cocker spaniels, and black-and-tan coonhounds. The hemorrhagic conditions observed with hemophilia B are similar to those observed with hemophilia A. Hemorrhagic conditions are often less pronounced in B than in A, but B may also be severe. Like hemophilia A the size of the dog has an influence on the expression of the condition, and bleeding is usually more severe in larger breeds. Some have reported that in hemophilia B, heterozygous females have a tendency to bleed.

PATHOPHYSIOLOGY. Factor IX, like factor VIII, is involved in the formation of the intrinsic prothrombin activator. This factor (factor IX) forms a complex with factor X. Some have stated that the factor IX defect arises from an abnormality of the prothrombin molecule, factor IX acting as an intermediate in the autocatalytic conversion of prothrombin to thrombin.

The hemophilia B disorder can be distinguished from that of hemophilia A in that B can be corrected with normal aged serum (which contains IX, but not factor VIII activity), whereas A can be corrected only with plasma.

INHERITANCE AND RECOMMENDATION. Like hemophilia A, hemophilia B is a sex-linked recessive trait, with the gene that allows bleeding located on the X chromosome.

See section for hemophilia A. To test for the heterozygous condition, mate females with a defective male. One defective pup proves the bitch heterozygous. Five nondefective male pups proves her homozygous dominant at the 95% level.

Factor VII Deficiency

A factor VII deficiency is found most often in the beagle but also has been reported in the Alaskan malamute. Clinical expression of the deficiency is usually mild, and a tendency for bleeding is usually not observed. The animals do bruise easily, and difficulty could be encountered following surgery or trauma. Dogs with this defect are reported to be very susceptible to demodectic mange due to a secondary moist tissue environment of the skin.

PATHOPHYSIOLOGY. Thromboplastin is the tissue extract that initiates the formation of the extrinsic prothrombin activator and interacts with several clotting factors. Factor VII is one of these. It is involved in the activation of factor X. In its absence the clotting defect is observed.

INHERITANCE AND RECOMMENDATION. The mode of inheritance suggested for the factor VII deficiency is an incompletely autosomal dominant.

If the trait is dominant, or incompletely dominant, removal of the affected animals should eliminate the trait. Also, apparently the heterozygotes can be detected by prothrombin times so they could also be removed from the breeding program.

Factor XI Deficiency (PTA)

A factor XI deficiency has been found in springer spaniels and Great Pyrenees. Minor bleeding episodes, such as hematuria (blood in urine) and subcutaneous hematomas (bleeding under the skin) are observed. Postsurgical bleeding (usually occurs within 24 hours) varies from severe to lethal.

PATHOPHYSIOLOGY. Factor XI is involved in the intrinsic clot mechanism. Dogs with the defect have less than 10% of the normal amounts of factor XI. The heterozygote has 25%–60% of the normal value.

INHERITANCE AND RECOMMENDATION. Factor XI defect is believed to be inherited as an incompletely autosomal dominant trait.

Procedures described to eliminate the factor VII deficiency defect could also be followed for factor XI.

Factor X Deficiency

A factor X deficiency has been reported in the cocker spaniel. The severity of bleeding in this breed varies. The disease is characterized by a high incidence of stillborn pups, and bleeding problems in the neonate can be severe to lethal. There may be bleeding from the umbilicus, mouth, and rectum; bruising of the skin; and massive intra-abdominal or intrathoracic bleeding. Pups may live up to 2 weeks of age and then fade or die suddenly. In mature dogs it is a clinically mild disease.

PATHOPHYSIOLOGY. Factor X, along with factor V, is involved in both the intrinsic and extrinsic systems. Factors X, V, and PF-3 (platelets) are concerned with the final step in prothrombin activator formation. Mild to moderate defects are observed in both extrinsic clotting (prothrombin and Russell's viper venom times) and intrinsic clotting (partial thromboplastin time), but platelet function and bleeding time are normal. Factor X activity varies from 18% to 65% of normal.

INHERITANCE. The trait is inherited as an incompletely autosomal dominant trait and may be lethal in the homozygous state. Tests suggest that affected animals surviving to maturity may be heterozygotes.

Von Willebrand's Disease (VWD)

A condition similar to Von Willebrand's disease in humans has been found for the most part in the German shepherd, golden retriever, miniature schnauzer, Doberman pinscher, and Scottish terrier.

Affected dogs exhibit mild to severe bleeding diathesis (tendency to leak blood from vessels), recurrent shifting lameness with radiographic changes similar to eosinophilic panosteitis, hematuria, recurrent diarrhea (usually stress induced) and melena (dark stools), chronic serosanguineous otitis externa (serum and blood from the ear), prolonged estrual and postpartum bleeding, and subcutaneous hematomas. Pups may be stillborn or fade early in life (within several days). Affected dogs are prone to mucous membrane bleeding. The disease becomes less severe with increasing age and repeated pregnancies.

PATHOPHYSIOLOGY. The disease is in some ways similar to hemophilia A since dogs with VWD also have a deficiency of factor VIII. VWD dogs have a low platelet retention (adhesiveness) and prolonged bleeding time. Intrinsic clotting times are abnormal but not to the extent observed in hemophilia A. Platelet aggregation and clot retraction are normal. Distinction between hemophilia A and VWD can be made. With VWD one observes reduced levels of both factor VII procoagulant activity and factor VIII–related antigen. In hemophilia A one finds a low factor VIII activity but normal or increased levels of factor VIII–related antigen.

INHERITANCE AND RECOMMENDATION. Incomplete autosomal dominant inheritance with variable expression is suggested for VWD. The heterozygous state may be clinically expressed as a more mild to moderate bleeding tendency.

Select against the trait as described above in hemophilia for dominant (by eliminating all affected animals) or incompletely dominant (by testing suspected animals) where possible to determine if they are heterozygous.

Fibrinogen Deficiency (Afibrinogenemia, Hypofibrinogenemia) (Fibrinogen Reduced or Absent)

Congenital deficiencies of fibrinogen (factor I) have been reported in dogs (collies and Saint Bernards). The dogs have a low level of plasma fibrinogen.

Affected individuals manifest a severe bleeding tendency and most do not survive beyond the neonatal stage. The most commonly observed problems are umbilical bleeding, recurrent hemarthrosis, and bleeding into the mucous membranes and subcutaneous tissues. The heterozygous state is usually revealed by subnormal fibrinogen levels.

PATHOPHYSIOLOGY. Fibrinogen is needed in the final stage of blood clotting. Fibrinogen is converted by thrombin to fibrin, which is essential for clot formation.

Bioassays for thrombin-responsive proteins are abnormal. Erythrocyte sedimentation and plasma viscosity are reduced as they depend on plasma fibrinogen concentration.

INHERITANCE AND RECOMMENDATION. Hypofibrinogenemia appears to be inherited as an incomplete dominant.

Select against this trait, as previously described for incompletely dominant genes.

Platelet Function Defects (Thrombopathia, Thrombasthenia)

Inherited defects of platelet function have been reported in the otter hound, foxhound, basset, and Scottish terrier. Each platelet defect has its own special characteristics. In the otter hound the defect appears to be a combination of thrombasthenic (functional deficiency) and thrombopathic (disturbance of platelet forming function) defects. In the basset it is thrombopathia. Mild to severe bleeding occurs in the homozygote with clinical signs mild or lacking in the heterozygote. The most common signs are hemarthrosis, bleeding from surface abrasions, and epithelial membrane bleeding (melena, gingival bleeding, hematuria, prolonged estrual discharge).

PATHOPHYSIOLOGY. Many of the tests of platelet function are abnormal. One observes prolonged bleeding times, normal or slightly reduced platelet counts, reduced platelet retention (adhesiveness), variable defects of aggregation, clot retraction, whole blood clotting time, prothrombin consumption time, and Russell's viper venom time. The latter abnormality, if present, results from a defect in platelet phospholipid activity.

INHERITANCE AND RECOMMENDATION. These defects appear to result from an incompletely autosomal dominant gene action.

Eliminate the gene from the kennel as described above for the type of gene action.

REFERENCES

Archer, R. K., and R. S. T. Bowden. 1959. A case of true hemophilia in a Labrador dog. Vet. Rec. 71:560–61.

Aufderheide, W. M., S. F. Skinner, and J. J. Kaneko. 1975. Clearance of cryoprecipitated factor VIII in canine hemophilia A. Am. J. Vet. Res. 36:367–70.

Bellars, A. R. M. 1969. Hereditary disease in British Antarctic sled dogs. Vet. Rec. 85:600–607.

_____. 1971. Genetic defects in Antarctic dogs. J. Small Anim. Pract. 12:493–500.

Bhatnagor, M. K., and S. Yamashuo. 1974. Parathyroid cytology of the hemophiliac dog. Anat. Histol. Embryol. 3:372.

Brinkhous, K. M., and J. B. Graham. 1950. Hemophilia in the female dog. Science. 3:723 24.

Brinkhous, K. M., P. D. Davis, J. B. Graham, and W. J. Dodds. 1973. Expression and linkage of genes for X-linked hemophilia A and B in the dog. Blood 41:577–85.

Brock, W. E., R. G. Buckner, J. W. Hampton, R. M. Bird, and C. E. Wulz. 1963. Canine hemophilia. Arch. Pathol. 76:464–69.

Brown, R. C., M. C. Swanton, and K. M. Brinkhous. 1963. Canine hemophilia and male pseudo-hermaphroditism cytogenic studies. Lab. Invest. 12:961–67.

Buckner, R. G., J. M. Hampton, R. M. Bird, and W. E. Brock. 1967. Hemophilia in the vizsla. J. Small Anim. Pract. 8:511–19.

Dodds, W. J. 1967. Familial canine thrombocytopathy. Thromb. Diath. Haemorrh. Suppl. 26:241–48.

_____. 1968. Current concepts of hereditary coagulation disorders in dogs. Exp. Anim. 1:243–59.

_____. 1970. Canine Von Willebrand's disease (hemophilia). J. Lab. Clin. Med. 76:713–21.

_____. 1971. Hemorrhagic disorders. In Current Veterinary Therapy. IV. Edited by Robert W. Kirk. Philadelphia: W. B. Saunders, pp. 247–54.

_____. 1973. Canine factor X (Stuart-Prower factor) deficiency. J. Lab. Clin. Med. 82:560–66.

_____. 1974. Blood coagulation, hemostasis, and thromboses. In A Handbook of Laboratory Animal Science. Edited by E. C. Melby, Jr., and N. H. Altman. Cleveland: Chemical Rubber Co., pp. 85–116.

_____. 1974. Hereditary and acquired hemorrhagic disorders in animals. In Progress in Hemostasis and Thrombosis. Edited by T. H. Spaet. New York: Grune and Stratton, vol. 2, pp. 215–47.

_____. 1975. Further studies of canine Von Willebrand's disease. Blood 45:221–30.

_____. 1975. Inherited hemorrhagic disorders. JAAHA 11:366–73.

_____. 1976. Inherited bleeding disorders. Purebred Dogs 93:31–38.

Dodds, W. J., M. A. Packham, H. C. Rowsell, and J. F. Mustard. 1967. Factor VII survival and turnover in dogs. Am. J. Physiol. 213:36–42.

Field, R. A., C. G. Richard, and F. B. Hutt. 1946. Hemophilia in a family of dogs. Cornell Vet. 36:285–300.

Graham, J. B., J. A. Buckwalter, L. J. Hartley, and K. M. Brinkhous. 1949. Canine hemophilia observations on the course: The clotting anomaly and the effect of blood transfusions. J. Exp. Med. 90:97–111.

Guyton, A. C. 1971. Textbook of Medical Physiology, 4th ed. Philadelphia: W. B. Saunders.

Hall, D. E. 1972. Blood Coagulation and Its Disorders in the Dog. Baltimore: Williams & Wilkins.

Hampton, J. W., R. G. Buckner, C. G. Cunn, L. R. Miller, and J. S. Mayes. 1973. Canine hemophilia in beagles: Genetics, site of factor VII synthesis and attempts at experimental therapy. Proc. 7th Congr. World Found. Haemophilia, May 17–20, 1971. Tehran Excerpta Med., pp. 26–32.

Hovig, T., H. C. Rowsell, W. J. Dodds, L. Jorgensen, and J. F. Mustard. 1967. Experimental hemostasis in normal dogs and dogs with congenital disorders of blood coagulation. Blood 30:363–668.

Kammermann, B., J. Gmur, and H. Stunzi. 1971. Afibrinogenamie bein Hund. Zentralbl. Veterinaermed. A. 18:192–205.

Kaneko, J. J., D. R. Cordy, and G. Carlson. 1967. Canine hemophilia resembling classic hemophilia A. JAVMA 150:15–21.

Lutz, F., S. Crane, and H. G. Downie. 1972. A study of a specific congenital platelet functional abnormality in dogs. In Program of 3rd Congr. Int. Soc. Thromb. Haematol., Washington, D.C., p. 220.

Meyers, J. L., K. R. Pierce, G. M. Gowing, and R. J. Leonpaker. 1972. Hereditary factor VII deficiency in the beagle. Br. J. Haematol. 23:59–67.

Mustard, J. F., H. C. Rowsell, G. A. Robinson, T. D. Hoeksema, and H. G. Downie. 1960. Canine hemophilia B (Christmas disease). Br. J. Haematol. 6:256–66.

Mustard, J. F., D. Secord, T. D. Hooksema, and H. G. Downie. 1962. Canine factor VII deficiency. Br. J. Haematol. 9:42–47.

Rowsell, H. C. 1963. Hemorrhagic disorders in dogs: Their recognition, treatment, and importance. Gaines Vet. Symp. (New Knowledge about Dogs) 12:9–16.

———. 1968. The hemostatic mechanism in mammals and birds in health and disease. Adv. Vet. Sci. 12:337–411.

Rowsell, H. C., H. G. Downie, J. F. Mustard, J. E. Leeson, and J. A. Archibald. 1960. A disorder resembling hemophilia B (Christmas disease) in dogs. JAVMA 137:247–50.

Sharp, A. A., and G. W. R. Dike. 1964. Hemophilia in the dog: Treatment with heterologous anti-hemophilia. Thromb. Diath. Haemorrh. 10:494–501.

Slappendel, R. J. 1975. Hemophilia A and hemophilia B in a family of French bulldogs. Tijdschr. Diergeneeskd. 100:20, 1075–88.

Spurberg, N. W., L. K. Burton, R. Peacock, and T. Pilling. 1972. Hereditary factor VII deficiency in the beagle. Br. J. Haematol. 23:59–67.

Wurzel, H. A., and W. C. Lawrence. 1961. Canine hemophilia. Thromb. Diath. Haemorrh. 6:98–103.

CANINE CYCLIC NEUTROPENIA

The gray collie syndrome (canine cyclic neutropenia) is a cyclic neutropenia in collie dogs associated with a specific dilution of hair color. Affected pups may be recognized at birth due to color; they are lethargic and may not suckle properly. Abscesses in the umbilical area may form and spread to other areas. The pups seldom live more than a few days, but on occasion they will survive 3–4 months and, with careful treatment, some may live 1 or 2 years.

The cyclic depression of circulating neutrophils occurs in affected collies every 10–11 days and lasts approximately 3 days. Cycles may begin as early as 1 week of age. Pups that survive at birth may do well for a short period (6 weeks) due to the presence of other immune mechanisms. Following the neutropenic phases one may observe episodes of fever, diarrhea, gingivitis, respiratory infection, lymphadenitis, and lameness due to bone necrosis. Dogs living past 4 months of age usually show amyloid deposition in the visceral organs and lymphoid tissue. Growth and sexual development are retarded. During the neutropenic episodes the dogs are susceptible to a wide range of bacterial and fungal infections. Clinical signs of infection usually subside 1–3 days following neutrophil repopulation. Even with clinical treatment dogs eventually develop lymphoid exhaustion, reticuloendothelial hyperplasia with monocytosis, anemia, and amyloidosis. Death usually results from secondary infections.

Pathophysiology

Cyclic neutropenia is a periodic, regularly recurring failure of cell maturation or an abnormality in the production of neutrophils in the bone marrow, apparently due to a defect in bone marrow cell differentiation or proliferation. A bone marrow hemopoietic defect, it occurs at a very early point in maturation, possibly at the level of differentiation from the stem cell (pluripotential stem cell with alternating competitive pressure). It is reflected as a complete suppression of the neutrophilic series from the myeloblast to the mature neutrophils or it indicates a lack of amplification in the myelocyte compartment. The production of both red and white blood cells (monocyte, lymphocyte, eosinophil, platelet, reticulocyte) is interrupted but, due to the comparatively long life of the red blood cell, this interruption is not as readily observed. The canine neutrophil has an average life span of 10 hours, so that when neutrophil production ceases, a rapid depletion is observed in the bone marrow reserve of segmented neutrophils followed by neutropenia.

Bone marrow recovery begins at a primitive stage with maturation proceeding in wavelike fashion through the neutrophil series. Large immature lymphocytes with intense basophilic cytoplasm are frequently observed during the neutropenic episodes and during the first few days after the return of the neutrophils to the peripheral blood. Monocytosis has been observed during the later portion of the neutropenic episode and for several days following. The bone marrow is hyperplastic and filled with megakaryocytes and myeloid cells in varying stages of maturity. Immature neutrophils predominate during the neutrophilic rebound phases.

Hemorrhage in and necrosis of the epiphyses of long bones are responsible for progressive lameness. Foci of necrosis are scattered throughout the bone marrow but are most common in the metaphysis and epiphyseal junction.

In the lymphoid system, the degree of lymphoid exhaustion and reticuloendothelial hyperplasia is directly related to length and severity of the disease. In lymph nodes of dogs surviving to adulthood, lymphocytes are depleted in paracortical areas and germinal centers are not seen.

Gray collies commonly are afflicted with ophthalmic lesions, and they have both microphthalmia and fundal ectasia. The latter is a herniation of the retinal and uveal layers of the eye through the sclera near the optic nerve. It appears through an ophthalmoscope as an elevation of the optic disc.

Amyloidosis occurs in dogs that have survived multiple episodes, preceded by increased levels and heterogeneity of serum globulins, particularly 2 globulin. All gonads are immature, the testes contain only spermatogonia, primary spermatocytes, and giant cells. Spermatids and mature sperm are absent. Ovaries contain primordial follicles with no evidence of mature or atretic follicles, corpora lutea, or corpora albicans.

The basis for the malabsorption part of the syndrome remains vague. In some dogs villi are short and crypts are elongated. The lamina propria is thickened and contains mononuclear inflammatory cells and neutrophils. Animals surviving to adulthood develop lymphoid exhaustion and reticuloendothelial hyperplasia. Monocytosis, anemia, and amyloidosis are seen in chronic cyclic neutropenia.

Inheritance

The gray collie syndrome is an inherited disease resulting from a simple autosomal recessive lethal gene. This disease has been observed only in collies. The gray color ranges from dark pewter gray to silver, dependent somewhat on the genotype of the parent stock. Pups with a genotype for sable tend to be light silver gray to dilute beige, while those of the tricolor genotype are deeper gray. A wavy coat of finer texture hair has been reported for affected pups.

It has not been determined if the phenotypically expressed dilute coat color and the blood abnormalities result from the same defective gene or if two linked genes are involved.

Gray color has been reported in the normal collie and is different from that observed in the gray collie syndrome. Both a recessive and a dominant type of gray color different from that observed in the gray collie syndrome have been reported.

Recommendation

Since the gray collie syndrome is the result of a recessive gene, elimination of affected dogs from the breeding program is not sufficient.

Selection against this gene requires the identification of the heterozygote that should not be included in future breeding programs. If the animal is of such value that the owner feels compelled to breed it, the consequences of such action need be understood, and all offspring tested.

A number of breeding tests may be used to identify carrier dogs. Since the gene is lethal, and the affected or homozygous recessive animals usually do not reach breeding age or attain puberty, these animals cannot be used for testing. This requires the use of the known carrier animals.

Since dogs have multiple births, one or two litters may be sufficient to test an individual.

Eleven normal offspring from a dog bred to known carriers of the recessive gene should give some assurance (95% of the time) that the dog being tested is free from the gene for gray collie syndrome. Sixteen normal offspring from a parent mated with known carriers suggest that 99% of the time the tested animal will not be a carrier. For the male, 24 normal and no defective pups from his own daughters would indicate an unaffected male.

REFERENCES

Adamson, J. W., D. C. Dale, and R. J. Elm. 1974. Regulation of cyclic erythropoiesis in the gray collie. J. Clin. Invest. 52:1A (abst.).

Cheville, N. F. 1968. Amyloidosis associated with cyclic neutropenia in the dog. Blood 31:111–14.

———. 1968. The gray collie syndrome. JAVMA 152:620–30.

———. 1975. The gray collie syndrome (cyclic neutropenia). JAAHA 11:350–52.

Cheville, N. F., R. C. Cutlip, and H. W. Moon. 1970. Microscopic pathology of the gray collie syndrome. Pathol. Vet. 7:225–45.

Dale, D. C., and R. G. Graw, Jr. 1974. Transplantation of allogeneic bone marrow in canine cyclic neutropenia. Science 183:83–84.

Dale, D. C., D. W. Alling, and S. M. Wolff. 1972. Cyclic hematopoiesis: The mechanism of cyclic neutropenia in gray collie dogs. J. Clin. Invest. 51:2197–2204.

Dale, D. C., S. B. Ward, H. R. Kimball, and S. M. Wolff. 1972. Studies of neutrophil production and turnover in gray collie dogs with cyclic neutropenia. J. Clin. Invest. 51:2190–96.

Ford, L. 1958. Possible pleiotrophic effects of the "gray" gene in collie dogs. Proc. 10th Int. Congr. Genet. 2:83.

———. 1963. Serial blood slides of lethal gray collie pups. Mod. Vet. Pract. 44:52–53.

———. 1969. Heredity aspects of human and canine cyclic neutropenia. J. Hered. 60:293–99.

Hartman, P. E., and S. R. Suskind. 1969. Gene Action, 2nd ed. Englewood Cliffs: Prentice-Hall.

Jones, J. B., E. S. Jones, and R. D. Lange. 1974. Early-life hematologic values of dogs affected with cyclic neutropenia. Am. J. Vet. Res. 35:849–52.

Jones, J. B., R. D. Lange, and E. S. Jones. 1975. Cyclic hematopoiesis in a colony of dogs. JAVMA 166:365–67.

Jones, J. B., R. D. Lange, T. J. Yang, H. Vodopick, and E. S. Jones. 1975. Canine cyclic neutropenia: Erythropoietin and platelet cycles after bone marrow transplantation. Blood 45:213–19.

Lund, J. E. 1970. Cyclic neutropenia in man and dog. In Animal Models in Biomedical Research. III. Washington, D.C.: National Academy of Sciences.

Lund, J. E., and G. A. Padgett. 1973. Canine cyclic neutropenia. Comp. Pathol. Bull. 5(2):2 4.

Lund, J. E., G. A. Padgett, and R. L. Ott. 1967. Cyclic neutropenia in gray collies. Blood 29:452-61.

Lund, J. E., G. A. Padgett, and J. R. Gorham. 1970. Additional evidence on the inheritance of cyclic neutropenia in the dog. J. Hered. 61:47-49.

Patt, H. M., J. E. Lund, and M. A. Maloney. 1973. Cyclic hematopoiesis in gray collie dogs: A stem cell problem. Blood 42:873-84.

Reynold, H. Y., D. C. Dale, S. M. Wolff, and J. S. Johnson. 1971. Serum immunoglobulin levels in gray collies. Soc. Exp. Biol. Med. 136:574-77.

Werden, P. L., B. Robinett, T. C. Graham, J. Adamson, and R. Storb. 1974. Canine cyclic neutropenia: A stem cell defect. J. Clin. Invest. 53:950-53.

Windhorst, D. R., J. E. Lund, J. Decker, and I. Swatz. 1967. Intestinal malabsorption in the gray collie syndrome. Fed. Proc. 26:260 (abst.).

Yang, T. J., J. B. Jones, E. S. Jones, and R. D. Lange. 1974. Serum colony stimulating activity of dogs with cyclic neutropenia. Blood 44:41-48.

Congenital Hemolytic Anemia (Basenji)

Congenital hemolytic anemia is a familial chronic nonspherocytic hemolytic anemia that occurs in the basenji dog and has been reported in the beagle. Apparently this condition results from a deficiency of the enzyme pyruvate kinase, an enzyme involved in anaerobic glycolysis within the erythrocyte. The deficiency is inherited as an autosomal recessive. The anemia is severe, unremitting, and progressive. The condition is usually observed before the dog is 1 year of age, and without treatment, death usually occurs before the dog reaches 3 years of age. Clinical signs are varied. Usually dogs appear normal in general appearance, body weight, and growth rate. Affected dogs may have decreased activity and may be less tolerant to exercise. Pale mucous membranes and splenomegaly (enlargement of spleen) are present. Hematologic findings include lowered packed cell volume, marked reticulocytosis, increased erythrocyte fragility, shortened red blood cell (RBC) life span and bone marrow erythroid hyperplasia. The Coomb's test for autoimmune hemolytic anemia is negative. Spherocytes (small spherical red blood cells) are not present.

Pathophysiology

Since mature erythrocytes have no citric acid cycle, energy for erythrocyte metabolism must be obtained by anaerobic glycolysis. The abnormality (anemia) apparently is the result of a deficiency of pyruvate kinase (PK) in the erythrocyte. Pyruvate kinase is required as a catalyst for the conversion of phosphoenolpyruvate to pyruvate. When this reaction becomes significantly rate limiting, the conversion of glucose to lactate is impaired, and there is an increase in glycolytic intermediates and an eventual adenosine triphosphate (ATP) deficiency. The ATP produced is not sufficient for red cell survival, hence, a premature senescence of the erythrocytes results. The hemograms are not compatible with the hematologic features of chronic blood loss anemia (iron deficiency), i.e., microcytosis, hypochromasia, and minimal bone marrow response. The macrocytosis, hypochromasia, reticulocytosis, and large number of nucleated erythrocytes in the peripheral blood indicate a very active erythroid regeneration. Bone marrow aspirations from all affected dogs substantiate the observation on peripheral blood. Bone marrow samples have low myeloid:erythroid ratios due to erythroid hyperplasia. Abnormal cells are not found in aspirated samples and erythroid maturation is normal. Osmotic fragility might appear normal on fresh blood samples but RBC fragility and autohemolysis increase following incubation. Some 4%–11% of RBC from PK-deficient basenji appeared as spheres. The spicules are smooth, blunt projections located equidistant from each other, with variable height (spheroechinocytes). The other RBC from basenji with PK deficiency anemia were similar to those from reticulocyte-rich blood of anemic dogs without PK deficiency.

Postmortem changes observed include splenomegaly and a slightly enlarged liver that is mahogany in color with grayish yellow foci. Some enlargement of lymph nodes is observed. Histologically, the spleen and some lymph nodes are highly cellular due to lymphoid hyperplasia and extramedullary hematopoiesis. Hemosiderin is found in many locations within the spleen. The liver has numerous infiltrating or proliferating exogenous cells, primarily in the portal regions, sinusoids, and the centrilobular area. These cells are mostly undifferentiated mononuclear cells, but other types may be seen. Kupffer cell (hepatic sinusoidal lining cells) hyperplasia and interlobular fibroplasia are seen. Hemosiderin is abundant in macrophages and sinusoidal endothelium. Lymphofollicular hyperplasia is a characteristic in all systemic nodes. The marrow spaces of the principal long bones are full of highly cellular red tissue, which indicates intense erythropoietic and granulopoietic activity.

Inheritance

Indications are that the hemolytic anemia syndrome is inherited clinically as a simple recessive. Apparently this condition is not related to sex and is not linked with coat color. However, since blood tests will allow the detection of carriers, because the heterozygote (carrier) has a measureable deficiency of PK, but still shows a phenotypically normal hemogram which indicates that one defective gene has a dosage effect (lowers the PK), some authors refer to the enzyme defect as codominant and the anemic condition as recessive.

Recommendation

Unless breeders are able to obtain an accurate PK deficiency test, they must rely on a breeding test to detect the carrier gene. PK deficiency tests are available. If sufficient normal carrier and anemic dogs are used to establish ranges, and if these tests are conducted by experienced individuals, it may be possible to determine the genotype. However, if this condition truly results from a completely recessive gene, the phenotypic expression of the homozygous normal and heterozygote carrier should be comparable.

A recessive individual as well as known carriers could be used for a breeding test. Five normal pups sired by or born to an individual dog when mated to known anemic dogs would be strong evidence that the animal was not a carrier of the gene. Eleven pups would be required for determining the carrier of the gene when mating the unknown (animal being tested) to known carriers.

REFERENCES

Brown, R., and T. S. Teng. 1975. Studies of inherited pyruvate kinase deficiency in the basenji. JAAHA 11:362-65.

Chandler, F. W., K. W. Prasse, and C. S. Callaway. 1975. Surface ultrastructure of pyruvate-kinase erythrocytes in the basenji dog. Am. J. Vet. Res. 36:1477-80.

Evans, J. M., and R. C. Povey. 1973. Congenital hemolytic anemia in the basenjis. Vet. Rec. 92:164.

Ewing, G. O. 1969. Familial nonspherocytic hemolytic anemia of basenji dogs. JAVMA 154:503-7.

Mullis, J. 1973. Hemolytic anemia in England. The Basenji J., p. 5.

Prasse, K. W. 1973. Nonspherocytic hemolytic anemia in basenji dogs. Personal communications.

Prasse, K. W., D. Carouoor, E. Deutler, M. Walker, and W. D. Schall. 1975. Pyruvate kinase deficiency anemia with terminal myelofibrosis and osteosclerosis in a beagle. JAVMA 166:1170-75.

Searcy, G. P., D. R. Miller, and J. B. Tasker. 1971. Congenital hemolytic anemia in the basenji dog due to erythrocyte pyruvate kinase deficiency. Con. J. Comp. Med. 35:67-70.

Tasker, J. B. 1970. Canine research today. Anim. Cavalcade (Winter), 1, 2, 12, 16, 21.

Tasker, J. B., G. A. Severin, S. Young, and E. J. Gillette. 1969. Familial anemia in the basenji dog. JAVMA 154:158-65.

Congenital Hemolytic Anemia (Alaskan Malamute)

An inherited macrocytic hemolytic anemia (and chondrodysplasia) is found in the Alaskan malamute. The anemia and short-limbed dwarfism are inherited as a pleitropic effect of a single gene. The chondrodysplasia is characterized by impaired growth of the bones in which one observes a delayed endochondral ossification. There is a gross thickening of the growth plate without loss of regular columns of cartilage cells but with apparent impairment of conversion of cartilage to bone.

Pathophysiology

The anemia is characterized by stomatocytosis, erythrocyte macrocytosis, low mean corpuscular hemoglobin concentration, increased osmotic fragility, shorter RBC life, reticulocytosis, erythroid hyperplasia and increased Fe turnover, mild anemia, and splenomegaly. No evidence of an effect on the white blood cell or platelet has been detected. Red cell survival is decreased in affected dogs. The anemia is characterized by stomatocytosis and increased red blood cell size (elevated mean corpuscular volume, decreased mean hemoglobin concentration, accompanied by normal absolute amount of red cell hemoglobin). Serum iron (abnormal hematocrit-hemoglobin ratio), B_{12}, and folate levels are normal. The red cell sodium is increased in affected dogs while the percent of solids is decreased. Studies indicate an increased transfer of sodium across the erythrocyte membrane, suggesting that the hemolytic disease is due to a defective (leaky) membrane or a defective ion transport mechanism that does not involve the cation-stimulated ATPase-mediated pump. The leaky membrane would result in the canine red cell Na pump attempting to compensate for the defect. The defect is intrinsic to the red cell and not to the reticuloendothelial system. The defective cells have a decreased life span.

From the skeletal standpoint, prominent features include marked widening of the zone of cartilage transformation; erythroid hyperplasia of the bone marrow; and abundant deposition of iron in kidney, spleen, and liver. Embden-Meyerhof enzyme deficiencies have not been observed.

Inheritance and Recommendation

Clinically the defect is expressed as an autosomal recessive. Certain hematologic parameters show that the heterozygote can be detected, so from this standpoint the condition appears to be incompletely dominant. RBC survival is normal in the heterozygote, and chondrodysplasia is not present. Red cell sodium concentration and water content are increased in anemic dogs and to a lesser extent in carriers.

Remove affected animals from the kennel. Test mate or have blood studies conducted to determine carriers.

REFERENCES

Fletch, S. M., and P. H. Pinkerton. 1972. An inherited anemia associated with hereditary chondrodysplasia in the Alaskan malamute. Can. Vet. J. 13:270–71.
———. 1973. Animal model of human disease: Congenital hemolytic anemia: Inherited hemolytic anemia with stomatocytosis in the Alaskan malamute dog. Am. J. Pathol. 71:477–80.
Fletch, S. M., M. C. Smart, P. W. Pennock, and R. E. Subden. 1973. Clinical and pathologic feature of chondrodysplasia (dwarfism) in the Alaskan malamute. JAVMA 162:357–61.
Fletch, S. M., P. H. Pinkerton, and P. J. Brueckner. 1975. The Alaskan malamute chondrodysplasia (dwarfism-anemia) syndrome in review. JAAHA 11:353–61.
Pinkerton, P. H., and S. M. Fletch. 1972. Inherited haemolytic anemia with dwarfism in the dog. Blood 40:963 (abst.).
Pinkerton, P. H., S. M. Fletch, P. J. Brueckner, and D. R. Miller. 1974. Hereditary stomatocytosis with hemolytic anemia in the dog. Blood 44(4):557–67.

Sande, R. D., J. E. Alexander, and G. Van Hoosier. 1970. Vitamin D resistant rickets in the malamute. Fed. Proc. 29:283 (abst.).

Sande, R. D., J. E. Alexander, and G. A. Padgett. 1974. Dwarfism in the Alaskan malamute: Its radiographic pathogenesis. J. Am. Vet. Radiol. Soc. 15:10–17.

Smart, M. C., and S. M. Fletch. 1971. A hereditary skeletal growth defect in purebred Alaskan malamutes. Can. Vet. J. 12:31–32.

Subden, R. E., S. M. Fletch, M. A. Smart, and R. G. Brown. 1972. Genetics of the Alaskan malamute chondrodysplasia syndrome. J. Hered. 63:149–52.

CONGENITAL HEREDITARY LYMPHOEDEMA

An inherited congenital lymphoedema has been traced to one poodle–labrador retriever cross. Clinically, one observes swollen (nonpainful) extremities and occasionally edema of the head, trunk, tail, etc. Edema usually is bilateral but not necessarily symmetrical. Edema usually decreases with age. Pups with an extreme case of lymphoedema may die during the neonatal period, with death resulting from secondary causes such as inability to nurse. Edema usually decreases with age.

Pathophysiology

This condition results from an abnormal development of the peripheral lymphatic system, including certain regional lymph nodes. There is an apparent failure of the central and peripheral lymphatic vessels to make an adequate connection, which results in improper lymphatic drainage. Absence of or hypoplasia of certain lymph nodes (popliteal, axillary), accompanied by dilation of the lymphatic vessels, is often observed.

Inheritance and Recommendation

This condition results from an autosomal dominant gene, with variable expressivity.

Since this condition results from a dominant gene and animals with the condition can be detected early, the trait may be eliminated simply by removing affected animals from a breeding program.

REFERENCES

Luginbuhl, H., S. K. Chocko, D. F. Patterson, and W. Medway. 1967. Congenital hereditary lymphoedema in the dog. Part II. Pathological studies. J. Med. Genet. 4:153–65.

Patterson, D. F., and W. Medway. 1966. Hereditary disease of the dog. JAVMA 149:1741–54.

Patterson, D. F., W. Medway, H. Luginbuhl, and S. Chocko. 1967. Congenital hereditary lymphoedema in the dog. Part I. Clinical and genetic studies. J. Med. Genet. 4:145–52.

CHAPTER 3

Cardiovascular System

At least twenty-two different congenital defects of the cardiovascular system have been reported for the dog. The incidence of any one of these may be low, but when combined these congenital defects may approach 10% of the observed heart diseases. In one report the rate of congenital heart disease in dogs presented to a university clinic was 6.8 per 1,000 while in another report the figure was approximately 47 per 1,000 dogs observed. It should be pointed out that these percentages might be somewhat inaccurate, since many pups affected may die before examination. Frequently, certain defects appear in combination with others. The congenital lesions most commonly reported in the literature and the percentage of each in three literature reviews and surveys are as follows: patent ductus arteriosus, 13.0%–31.0%; pulmonic stenosis, 8.3%–17.6%; aortic stenosis, 3.0%–5.1%.

These above-listed defects account for approximately 70% of all congenital heart defects.

The facts that congenital defects are three times more common in the purebred dog (8.9/1,000) than in dogs of mixed breeding (2.6/1,000) and that these defects occur more frequently in certain breeds are suggestive of a genetic predisposition. However, one must consider the percentages of purebred dogs versus mixed dogs presented.

PATENT DUCTUS ARTERIOSUS (PDA)

Prior to birth, the vast majority of an animal's blood bypasses the lungs and flows from the right ventricle and pulmonary trunk through the ductus arteriosus, a short vascular connection, to the aortic arch and thus to systemic circulation. At birth, or very soon thereafter (24 hours), the ductus arteriosus functionally closes. Closure occurs in two phases. The first phase, a functional closure only, is initiated by a change in oxygen tension. The second phase, complete anatomical closure, occurs over a period of time. If functional closure does not occur, and the ductus remains open or patent after the first few hours or days following birth, it is considered to be an anomaly and is called a patent ductus arteriosus (PDA).

Two clinically recognizable types of PDA may be observed: one, a PDA with a left to right shunt, and the other, PDA with a right to left shunt and severe pulmonary hypertension. With a left to right shunt, the pup appears normal at first, will have normal heart sounds, and will make normal increases in weight. Then, between the 2nd and 14th days of life, a systolic or transystolic murmur may be detected. By the 2nd or 3rd week the murmur becomes continuous, increases in loudness, and may be accompanied by a palpable precordial thrill (a turbulence within the vessel). Left heart failure occurs in a large proportion of the affected pups between the 2nd and 5th weeks. Rapid labored breathing, weight loss, and pulmonary rales are evident. If the pup survives this period, it will usually reach adulthood. Long-term survival is not expected. The dog may exhibit fatigue and show a lack of stamina, dyspnea (difficulty in breathing), hind limb weakness, weight loss, abdominal swelling, coughing after exercise, and occasional fainting.

Less frequently observed are the cases of PDA with a right to left shunt and pulmonary hypertension. Here, pulmonary arterial pressure in the pulmonary trunk is equal to or greater than that of the aorta. The result is cardiac overloading and right ventricular hypertrophy. Caudal (back portion of body) cyanosis (poor oxygenation of tissues) may be observed.

A murmur may be heard early in life but usually disappears. The second heart sound becomes accentuated and split. If not detected when the dog is a pup, visible signs of the defect may not appear until later in life when noticeable signs such as weakness of the rear legs following exercise is exhibited.

Pathophysiology

Research indicates that in the PDA pup the abnormality concerns the vessel wall structure and the ability of the ductus to undergo functional closure. Apparently there is a deficiency and/or abnormal distribution of the smooth muscle in the ductus arteriosus. PDA pups also have a decreased rate of ductus arteriosus degeneration and an increased amount of elastic tissue with asymmetrical distribution of both muscle and elastic tissue elements. Histologically, the affected segment resembles that of the non-contractile portion of the aorta. Variation in the expression of the trait probably results from the variation in the quantity of affected tissue.

Inheritance and Recommendation

A predisposition to PDA has been suggested for the toy and miniature poodles, the Pomeranian, collie, cocker spaniel, and Shetland sheepdog. The condition does occur, of course, in other breeds. Some evidence indicates a greater frequency in the female. Recent studies and the variation of the expression of PDA indicate a polygenic (multiple or additive) type of inheritance, a threshold trait of very high heritability. It appears that a dog with intermediate expression of the trait mentioned above transmits it to the same extent as one with a greater phenotypic expression of the trait. That is, the genes involved act additively to produce increasing liability to defective development, with discrete anatomic defects occurring at critical thresholds on the underlying scale. The larger the "dose" of gene, the more severe the defect.

One should not use affected dogs or dogs closely related to affected dogs for breeding.

PULMONIC STENOSIS

Pulmonic stenosis is a narrowing or obstructing of the opening between the right ventricle and pulmonary trunk. Often the obstruction is due to the fusion of the valve cusps (leaves), which results in an opening of reduced size, but the condition may also result from the formation of a fibrous ring immediately below the valve or a muscular narrowing of the ventricular outflow.

Many of the dogs with this condition do not show any noticeable clinical symptoms but upon examination reveal a characteristic systolic murmur. In pups with a severe condition and in some adults, dyspnea, tiring during exercise, fainting, and right heart failure are observed. Venous congestion and ascites (fluid accumulation in abdomen) may also be observed. Affected dogs usually do not live past 3 years of age.

The defect is reported to occur most frequently in the English bulldog, Chihuahua, fox terrier, Samoyed, beagle, and schnauzer.

Pathophysiology

This defect may often be present with other defects. Four types are reported: (1) subvalvular (the most common), a fibrous band just below the valve, (2) valvular obstruction at the valve proper, (3) supravalvular obstruction (very rare) in the pulmonary trunk, and (4) infundibular or muscular stenosis in the right ventricular outflow tract.

Inheritance and Recommendation

Studies as to the inheritance of pulmonic stenosis have not been extensive. Reports from those most knowledgeable indicate this condition is inherited in a similar manner to PDA (polygenic, threshold trait).

The recommendation is the same as for PDA.

AORTIC STENOSIS

Aortic stenosis is a narrowing or a constriction in the left ventricular outflow channel at the aortic valve region.

Aortic stenosis is most frequently observed in the German shepherd and boxer but has been found in other breeds such as the English bulldog, fox terrier, Newfoundland, and springer spaniel. Pups may appear to be of normal health. In the more severe cases, coughing and dyspnea may be observed (left heart involvement). Limb edema and ascites (right heart problem) may be noticed in advanced cases. Syncope (fainting) and death may occur.

Pathophysiology

Three distinct types of aortic stenosis are mentioned in the literature. The most common of the three is subvalvular (subaortic) in which there is a fibrous ring (of various degrees) located in the left ventricular outflow tract below the aortic valve. The other two types—valvular aortic stenosis and the supravalvular type—are rare. The fibrous connective tissue reduces blood flow from the left ventricle to the aorta. This results in a turbulent blood flow and a systolic murmur. An enlargement of the left ventricle results.

Also noted are extensive lesions of the intramural branches of the coronary arteries and focal infarction (clots) and fibrosis of the left ventricular myocardium.

Inheritance and Recommendation

The genetic pattern is believed to be similar to that outlined for PDA. Likewise similar recommendations for eliminating the gene are in order.

ATRIAL SEPTAL DEFECT

An atrial septal defect refers to an opening or hole in the atrial septum, the tissue that divides the left and right atria. More often than not the defect will be associated with some other form of heart defect. The defect may be one of three types, two of which are true interatrial defects. One, an ostium primum defect, occurs when the defect is in the lower portion of the septum and no tissue is found between the defect and the atrioventricular valve. This condition is much less frequent than the second type, ostium secundum, with the defect in the upper to the middle portion; the third type would be a patent foramen ovale (persistent opening or failure of normal closure). Clinical signs include dyspnea, fatigue, weakness. Ascites may be present if the dog is in right-sided heart failure. An ejection murmur may be heard. Split heart sounds may be heard and auscultation of the lungs may reveal rales.

The condition frequently occurs in the boxer.

Physiopathology

The above defect causes the shunting of the blood from the left atrium to the right side or right atrium. This, of course, causes an increased volume of blood in the right atrium, resulting in an overload on the right side and in the lungs. The right atrium and right ventricle and the left atrium may enlarge, and pulmonary congestion may occur. If for some reason the blood pressure causes a right to left shunt, cyanosis may be observed.

An observed murmur may result from the other accompanying heart defects.

Inheritance and Recommendation

Limited findings suggest the same type of inheritance for atrial septal defect as for PDA and the same suggestion for eliminating the trait.

VENTRICULAR SEPTAL DEFECT

Ventricular septal defect is an opening between the ventricles, most frequently located near the lower portion of the septum.

If the opening in the septum is small, no symptoms may be observed. In any case the pup may not initially exhibit any symptoms. Occasional congestive heart failure is noted. Other signs may be fatigue, venous distention, and ascites. The Siberian husky appears to have a predisposition for this defect.

Pathophysiology

During the contraction of the heart, the higher pressure in the left heart shunts the blood from the left ventricle to the right ventricle. In so doing, a turbulent blood flow and a resultant systolic murmur are created. The blood volume overload on the right ventricle causes it to enlarge. If the left-right blood shunt is sufficient, pulmonary hypertension develops. It is possible the right ventricular pressure may increase until it equals that on the left side. This could cause the venous blood to be shunted into the systemic circulation, resulting in cyanosis.

Inheritance and Recommendation

Detailed genetic studies of ventricular septal defect are not available. Indications at present are that the mode of inheritance and the recommendations suggested for PDA, etc., are acceptable.

TETRALOGY OF FALLOT

Tetralogy of Fallot is a complex heart malformation found frequently in the keeshond.

This complex is composed of a high ventriclular septal defect, varying degrees of aortic overriding, and pulmonary stenosis. The fourth common feature of the complex is right ventricular hypertrophy, which occurs as a secondary defect.

This condition can often be detected as early as weaning age. A frequent sign would be the cyanotic pup, as well as stunting and shortness of breath. Signs may increase with age.

Pathophysiology

Various degrees of severity will be noted. In cases where pulmonic stenosis is moderate to severe, the right ventricular contraction pressure approaches or suppresses that of the left ventricle. A proportion of the right ventricle outflow then passes directly to the aorta without being oxygenated. This results in cyanosis. If the pulmonic stenosis is mild and the ventricular septal defect is small, the above pressure changes do not occur and one observes a left to right shunt. An affected dog would not be cyanotic.

Inheritance and Recommendation

The suggested mode of inheritance for tetralogy of Fallot is complex; and a single gene with modifiers has been suggested by some while others suggest a polygenic (additive) trait as for PDA.

Recommended genetic correction would be as outlined for other heart defects.

PERSISTENT RIGHT AORTIC ARCH

Persistent right aortic arch is a vascular ring abnormality that results in a constriction of the esophagus and on occasion the constriction of the trachea. This condition is due to the aorta orginating from the right fourth aortic arch instead of the left fourth aortic arch. With the aorta going to the right of the esophagus, the ligamentum arteriosum forms the dorsolateral aspect on the right (or left dorsolateral), the pulmonary artery on the left, and the base of the heart the ventral aspect of the ring, thereby encircling the esophagus.

The defect is usually first noticed when the pup begins to eat solid food. Soon after eating, the pup may regurgitate or vomit due to failure of the food to pass through the esophagus. This leads to emaciation, increased appetite, dehydration, stunted pups, and often aspiration pneumonia. While eating, the dog may assume a posture of lowered head and straight neck in an attempt to straighten the esophagus and aid in swallowing. The condition is most common in Irish setters, German shepherds, and Boston terriers.

Pathophysiology

The defect results in the inability of the pup to properly swallow its food.

Inheritance and Recommendation

There are no specific data for this defect. It is considered by some to be similar to PDA.

REFERENCES

Buchanan, J. W., D. F. Patterson, and R. L. Pyle. 1971. Morphologic studies in dogs with hereditary patent ductus arteriosus. Circulation 53–54:147 (suppl. II, abstracts 44th Scientific Sessions, Am. Heart Assoc.).

Detweiler, D. K. 1964. Genetic aspects of cardiovascular diseases in animals. Circulation 30:114–27.

Ettinger, S. J., and P. F. Suter, consulting editor. 1970. Cardiovascular Diseases. Philadelphia: W. B. Saunders.

Eyster, G. E. 1972. Pulmonic stenosis. In A Manual of Clinical Cardiology. Am. Anim. Hosp. Assoc., pp. 37–40.

Flickinger, G. L., and D. F. Patterson. 1967. Coronary lesions associated with congenital subaortic stenosis in the dog. J. Pathol. Bacteriol. 93(1):133–40.

Kirk, R. W., editor. Veterinary Therapy. V. Philadelphia, London, Toronto. W. B. Saunders, pp. 251–74.

Knauer, K. W. 1972. Interventricular septal defects. In A Manual of Clinical Cardiology. Am. Anim. Hosp. Assoc., pp. 23–28.

Knight, D. H., D. F. Patterson, and J. Melbin. 1971. Constriction of the fetal ductus arteriosus in normal dogs and those genetically predisposed to persistent patency. Circulation 53–54:114 (suppl. II, abstracts 44th Scientific Sessions, Am. Heart Assoc.).

Mulnix, J. A., and G. A. Severin. 1972. Persistent right aortic arch. In A Manual of Clinical Cardiology. Am. Anim. Hosp. Assoc., pp. 17–21.

Mulvihill, J. J. 1971. Comment on the epidemiology of congenital heart disease in dogs. Birth Defects: Original article series, Vol. VIII, Cardiovascular System. National Foundation. Paper presented at 4th Conference of Clinical Delineation of Birth Defects, Baltimore, Md., June 1971.

Patterson, D. F. 1965. Congenital heart disease in the dog. Ann. N.Y. Acad. Sci. 127:541–69.

_____. 1968. Epidemiologic and genetic studies of congenital heart disease in the dog. Circ. Res. 23:171–202.

_____. 1971. Canine congenital heart disease: Epidemiology and etiologic hypotheses. J. Small Anim. Pract. 12:263–87.

_____. 1972. Patent ductus arteriosus. In A Manual of Clinical Cardiology. Am. Anim. Hosp. Assoc., pp. 5–16.

_____. 1972. Tetralogy of Fallot. In A Manual of Clinical Cardiology. Am. Anim. Hosp. Assoc., pp. 41–46.

Patterson, D. F., and D. K. Detweiler. 1963. Predominance of German shepherd and boxer breeds among dogs with congenital subaortic stenosis. Am. Heart J. 65:249–430.

_____. 1967. Hereditary transmission of patent ductus arteriosus in the dog. Am. Heart J. 74:289–90.

Patterson, D. F., and W. Medway. 1966. Hereditary diseases of the dog. JAVMA, 149:1741–54.

Patterson, D. F., and R. L. Pyle. 1971. Genetic aspects of congenital heart disease in the dog. Proc. 21st Gaines Vet. Symp., pp. 20–28.

Patterson, D. F., R. L. Pyle, J. W. Buchanan, E. Trautvetter, and D. A. Abt. 1971. Hereditary patent ductus arteriosus and its sequelae in the dog. Circ. Res. 29:1–13.

Patterson, D. F., R. L. Pyle, and J. W. Buchanan. 1972. Hereditary cardiovascular malformations of the dog. Birth defects. Original article series, Vol. VIII, Cardiovascular System. National Foundation, pp. 160–74.

Pyle, R. L. 1972. Aortic stenosis. In A Manual of Clinical Cardiology. Am. Anim. Hosp. Assoc., pp. 25–35.

CHAPTER 4

Sensory Organs

EYE

Cataracts

The term *cataract* refers to an ocular condition, frequently observed in dogs, which results in a partial or total opacity of the crystalline lens or its capsule. Cataracts result from various causes, and the exact cause of a cataract observed in an individual dog is often difficult to determine. Cataracts may result from trauma, nutritional deficiencies, diabetes mellitus, etc., or may be congenital. Congenital cataracts may or may not be inherited. Cataracts may be primary or secondary. Primary cataracts are the type observed when no other ocular abnormality is present. Secondary cataracts are those that are associated with or accompany another eye disorder, such as generalized progressive retinal atrophy. This type of secondary cataract is frequently found in miniature and toy poodles and English cocker spaniels. Secondary cataracts occur in some cases of retinal dysplasia (abnormal retinal formation) described in Sealyhams, Bedling- tons, and Labrador retrievers. Persistent pupillary membrane in the basenji may be associated with nonprogressive cataracts. Dislocation of the lens is hereditary in fox terriers, Sealyham terriers, and Jack Russell terriers, and hereditary cataracts apparently have two different genetic forms. One is reported due to a dominant gene, perhaps with incomplete penetrance in some strains or breeds. Affected dogs usually show defective vision between 1 and 3 years of age. Breeds in which cataracts have been reported sug- gestive of a dominant type of inheritance include golden retrievers, Labrador retrievers, pointers, German shepherds, and beagles. The second form and the most frequent type in dogs apparently results from a simple

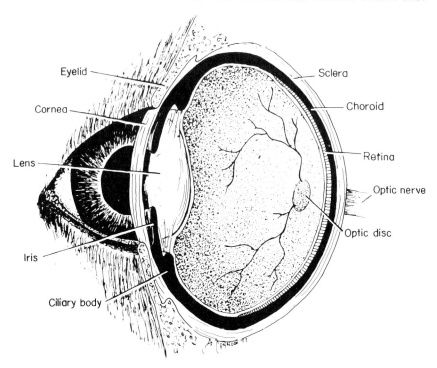

Fig. 4.1. *Diagram of the eye. Light energy transmitted through the pupil is deflected by the lens and the energy cast on the retina. This energy excites receptor cells in the retina and the impulse is transmitted to the brain for interpretation.*

autosomal recessive. This type usually occurs at a younger age than does the dominant type and progresses until the dog is completely blind, usually between 2 and 3 years of age. Predisposed breeds include Boston terriers, Staffordshire terriers, Old English sheepdogs, miniature schnauzers (recessive), cocker spaniels, poodles (recessive in standard), fox terriers, and Afghans (recessive). The incidence or frequency of occurrence of cataracts varies. It is also possible that both types of inheritance could occur within the same breed. In one study, 88% of the American cockers examined exhibited lenticular opacities of some degree, with 11% having mature to hypermature cataracts. In one survey of 291 Afghans, only 5 had cataracts. Cataracts were detected in 43 of 66 Old English sheepdogs presented to a specialty practice. In one group of adult golden retrievers prevalence of cataracts was 13.9%.

PATHOPHYSIOLOGY. The cataract due to a dominant gene is a posterior polar cataract appearing as an inverted Y or triangle, or irregular circle of opacity, at the pole, and not associated with the hyaloid artery. These cataracts show little tendency to progress until senile changes occur. Other types include cortical, cortical and polar, and total. These are usually, but not always, bilateral and symmetrical. Cortical cataracts progress and dogs show defective vision at 1-3 years of age. Congenital cataracts consistently reveal a posterior capsular deformity. In all instances the capsular defect in this condition appeared as a homogenous (hyaline) staining material lacking in continuity.

The recessive type cataracts are usually bilateral, symmetrical, and progressive. This type is observed earlier, first at a few months of age, and progresses until total and mature at 2-3 years of age. A cataract appears dense with flecks in the pupillary region, often roughly in the form of the suture lines. Cortical and peripheral opacities are also seen and the most dense part is in the nuclear region of the lens.

A secondary cataract may begin as a cortical type, often posterior with typical appearance of vacuoles (clear spaces) arranged in a wedge-shaped area from the periphery of the lens. These are progressive and ultimately mature to total opacity, thus not allowing examination of the retina for presence of retinopathy (retinal disease).

Factors indicating that progressive retinal atrophy was the primary condition included a poor pupillary light reflex; breed, age, and history of the development of poor vision; and night blindness.

INHERITANCE AND RECOMMENDATION. Two types of inheritance have been reported and described above, with breed and incidence reported where known.

Dominant and recessive forms of this condition should be tested for as described previously for this type of gene action, and positive breeding animals should be eliminated.

REFERENCES

Anderson, A. C., and F. T. Schultz. 1958. Inherited (congenital) cataract in the dog. Am. J. Pathol. 34:965-75.

Barnett, K. C. 1972. Types of cataract in the dog. JAAHA. 8:2-9.

Donovan, R. 1971. Congenital cataracts in the miniature schnauzer. Proc. Am. Coll. Vet. Ophthalmol. Las Vegas 2:36-46.

Gelatt, K. N. Oct. 1972. Cataracts in the golden retriever dog. Vet. Ophthalmol. Vet. Med. Small Anim. Clin., pp. 1113-15.

Greene, J. E. Winter 1953. Cataracts. Auburn Vet. 9(2):82-86.

Heywood, R. 1971. Juvenile cataracts in the beagle dog. J. Small Anim. Pract. 12:171-77.

Koch, S. A. 1972. Cataracts in interrelated Old English sheepdogs. JAVMA 160:299-301.

_____. 1972. Cataracts in Old English sheepdogs: A preliminary report. JAAHA 8:61-63.

Koch, S. A., and L. F. Rubin. 1967. Probably nonhereditary congenital cataracts in dogs. JAVMA 150:1374-76.

Magrane, W. G. 1971. Canine Ophthalmology, 2nd ed. Philadelphia: Lea & Febiger.

Olesen, H. P., O. A. Jensen, and M. S. Norn. 1974. Congenital hereditary cataract in cocker spaniels. J. Small Anim. Pract. 15:741-50.
Prester, W. A. 1972. Congenital ocular defects in cattle, horses, cats and dogs. JAVMA 160:1504-11.
Roberts, S. R. 1973. Hereditary cataracts. Vet. Clin. North Am. 3(3):433-37.
Roberts, S. R., and L. C. Helper. 1972. Cataracts in Afghan hounds. JAVMA 160:427-32.
Rubin, L. F. 1967. Clinical electroretinography in dogs. JAVMA 151:1456-69.
Rubin, L. F., and R. D. Flowers. 1972. Inherited cataract in a family of standard poodles. JAVMA 161:207-8.
Rubin, L. F., S. A. Koch, and R. J. Huber. 1969. Hereditary cataracts in miniature schnauzers. JAVMA 154:1456-58.
Startup, F. G. 1969. Diseases of the canine eye. Baltimore: Williams & Wilkins.
Yakely, W. L., G. A. Hegreberg, and G. A. Padgett. 1971. Familial cataracts in the American cocker spaniel. JAAHA 7:127-35.

Collie Eye Anomaly

The collie eye anomaly is an inherited congenital defect, which in its extreme results in blindness in the affected animal. This defect has been widespread in the collie and occurs also in Shetland sheepdogs. The literature suggests that at one time 80%-90% of collies were affected to some degree. A greatly decreased prevalence has resulted from selective breeding. This genetic defect occurs equally in both sexes and has been reported in both smooth and rough collies, as well as in sable and white, tricolors, whites, and blue merles. The defect is bilateral but not symmetrical, meaning that one eye of the affected individual may show different signs and degrees of the syndrome from those observed in the other eye.

The owner of the individual animal may not be aware that the animal is affected and may not present the animal for examination unless defective vision or the possible sudden appearance of blood in the eye is observed.

In the past, collie eye anomaly has been known as, or referred to as, congenital anomaly of the optic disc, congenital posterior ectasia of the sclera, collie ectasic syndrome, and ocular fundus anomaly. Microphthalmus, which is often observed in the collie and Shetland sheepdog, is not necessarily indicative of an affected eye.

PATHOPHYSIOLOGY. The percentage of affected dogs with defective vision is relatively small. Complete loss of vision occurs suddenly due to retinal detachment. One may observe intraocular hemorrhage in conjunction with or immediately following retinal detachment. Hemorrhage may also occur from bleeding of new vessels formed on the surface of the retina.

In one study the ocular defects observed, listed in order of frequency, were as follows:

Grade 1. Unusual tortuosity of the retinal arteries and veins. This condition may be present with no other obvious lesions or may be observed in eyes showing other lesions associated with the collie eye anomaly. The presence of these lesions alone does not necessarily condemn a dog, since some affected dogs have reasonably normal retinal vessels. A pale area (chorioretinal dysplasia) of variable size may be situated temporally and supratemporally from the optic disc.

Grade 2.   Congenital and nonprogressive. This condition may be slight or extensive. The choroidal pigment is poorly developed or may be absent. The large choroidal vessels are visible beneath the retinal vasculature. The sclera can usually be seen as a white background. The defect in the fundus is in the mesodermal component of the vascular and nonvascular tissue derived from the outer layer of the embryonic optic cup. This has been termed hypoplasia of the choroid, tapetum, and retina and is considered the hallmark of the abnormal collie fundus. Pits in or adjacent to the optic nerve head (defect known as coloboma) and ectasia of the optic disc are noted on examination with an ophthalmoscope. These pits appear to be gray blue or red and out of focus. The disc may appear larger than normal. Pits are usually situated at the temporal (dorsolateral) or inferior (lower) border, and vessels may not be visible ophthalmoscopically because they are out of focus. They are accompanied by the pale area mentioned above and are not always bilateral.

Grade 3.   Posterior scleral ectasia in the region of the optic nerve entrance (often with detachment of the retina), juxtapapillary or circumpapillary staphyloma (protrusion). This is the most severe form of the collie eye anomaly. This condition involves a large area of the posterior fundus including the optic nerve head that protrudes posteriorly by 5–35 dioptres (3 dioptres = 1 mm) and appears externally as a bluish blister like protrusion of the sclera. Often the optic disc is not visible by ophthalmoscopy. The posterior pole is poorly pigmented and ectatic and the optic nerve may be maldirected. Retinal blood vessels disappear over the edge of the area. This lesion is congenital, nonprogressive, and often bilateral.

Grade 4.   Retinal detachment. In the majority of cases, this occurs only in the most severely affected animals. Detachment may be congenital or occur shortly after birth and become expanded with time. Retinal detachment need not be bilateral.

Grade 5.   Hemorrhage.

INHERITANCE. Although some early reports suggested that the collie eye anomaly had a polygenic origin, it is now generally accepted that this syndrome (choroidal dysplasia) results from an autosomal recessive gene with variable expressivity. It has been suggested, but not confirmed nor widely accepted, that one manifestation of this syndrome, staphyloma, reportedly observed in 34% of the eyes examined in one study, is inherited independently as a dominant. Staphyloma, however, is consistently observed in connection with chorioretinal dysplasia.

The question of a possible relationship between coat color and ocular lesions must be considered. One must not confuse the natural appearance of the eye of the blue merle with the collie eye lesions. Also when discussing collie eye and coat color association one must be extremely careful to distinguish between the gene for merling and the gray-silver color exhibited with the gray collie syndrome. However, one cannot discount that the gene for merling or dappling (hereditary dilution of color, extreme when homozygous) is associated with a heterochromia of the iris in several species. Since chorioretinal dysplasia seen in collie eyes is associated with a lack of pigment in the choroid and retinal epithelium, one should not too lightly exclude the possibility that the eye lesions are linked in some way with the genes for color. It has been reported and confirmed that the tapetum is absent or rudimentary in color-dilute dogs. The gene for merling may be present but phenotypically masked in some coat colors.

RECOMMENDATION. Since the congenital condition can be detected at a relatively early age in puppies (as early as 3 weeks but with accuracy by 6 weeks of age), all puppies should be examined before they are sold, and the purchaser should be informed as to the condition of the individual dog.

All dogs that are to be considered for breeding stock should be reexamined at a later date.

Dogs with any degree or sign of this syndrome should not be used for breeding. Puppies have been produced with all degrees of defects from parent stock showing only a slight degree (Grade 1) of the syndrome.

Animals that appear normal should be tested by breeding to determine if they are carriers (heterozygous for the condition). One affected pup condemns both parents as carriers.

If the owner of an affected dog feels the animal is otherwise of such genetic worth that it must be used in his breeding program, the result of this action should be explained, and suggestions made as to breeding programs to follow.

REFERENCES

Barnett, K. C. 1965. Canine retinopathies. III. Other breeds. J. Small Anim. Pract. 6:185–96.
_____. 1967. Factors influencing official control of hereditary defect in dogs: Ophthalmological aspects. Proc. 18th World Vet. Congr., Paris 2:491–94.
_____. 1969. The collie eye anomaly. Vet. Rec. 84:431–34.
_____. 1969. Genetic anomalies of the posterior segment of the canine eye. J. Small Anim. Pract. 10:451–55.
Blogg, J. R. 1969. The normal and abnormal fundus in dog and cat. Victorian Vet. Proc. 27:45–47.
_____. 1970. Collie anomaly. Aust. Vet. J. 46:530–32.
Cello, R. M. 1969. Collie eye anomaly: Comments. JAVMA 155:870–71.
Cole, W. W. 1970. Breeding of collies with collie eye anomaly. (Letter). JAVMA 156:4.
Donovan, E. F., and M. Wyman. 1965. Ocular fundus anomaly in the collie. JAVMA 147:1465–69.

Donovan, R. H. 1965. Collie eye syndrome. Mod. Vet. Pract. 46(9):34 (abst.).

_____. 1965. Chorioretinal dysplasia, juxtapapillary staphyloma and retinal detachment in the collie. Proc. Am. Soc. Vet. Ophthalmol., Portland, 8–24.

Donovan, R. H., and A. M. MacPherson. 1968. The inheritance of chorioretinal dysplasia and staphyloma in the collie. Carnivore Genet. Newsletter 5:85–89.

Donovan, R. H., H. Mackenzie Freeman, and C. L. Schepens. 1969. Anomaly of the collie eye. JAVMA 155:872–75.

Fox, M. W. 1970. Inherited structural and functional abnormalities in the dog. Can. Vet. J. 11:5–12.

Freeman, H. M., R. H. Donovan, and C. L. Schepens. 1966. Retinal detachment, chorioretinal changes and staphyloma in the collie. I. Ophthalmoscopic findings. Arch. Ophthalmol. 76:412–21.

Gelatt, K. N., and L. A. Veith. 1970. Hereditary multiple ocular anomalies in Australian shepherd dogs. Vet. Med. Small Anim. Clin. 65:39–42.

Hallstrom, M. 1971. Collie eye anomaly. (Swedish) Sven. Vet. Tidn. 23:364–66.

Latshaw, W. K. 1968. A study of the prenatal stage of the collie eye anomaly. Ph.D. dissertation, Ohio State Univ.

Latshaw, W. K., M. Wyman, and W. G. Venzke. 1969. Embryologic development of an anomaly of ocular fundus in the collie dog. Am. J. Vet. Res. 30:211–17.

Lawson, D. D. 1968. The collie eye anomaly. (Letter.) Vet. Rec. 84:618.

Mackenzie, F. H., R. H. Donovan, and C. L. Schepens. 1969. Chorioretinal changes, juxtapapillary staphyloma, and retinal detachment in the collie. Bibl. Ophthalmol. 1969:111–17.

Magrane, W. 1953. Congenital anomaly of the optic nerve in collies. North Am. Vet. 34:646.

Mason, T. A., and K. Cox. 1971. Collie eye anomaly. Aust. Vet. J. 47:38–40.

Priester, W. A. 1972. Congenital ocular defects in cattle, horses, cats, and dogs. JAVMA 160:1504–11.

Roberts, S. R. 1960. Congenital eye defects in dogs. Purebred Dogs 77(9):14–15.

_____. 1961. Congenital posterior ectasia of the sclera in collies. Vet. Excerpts 21(3):63–67.

_____. 1964. Three inherited ocular defects in the dog. Mod. Vet. Pract. 48(2):30–34.

_____. 1967. Color dilution and hereditary defects in collie dogs. Am. J. Ophthalmol. 63:1762–75.

_____. 1968. Hereditary diseases of the eye in dogs: The collie ectasia syndrome. Vet. Scope 12:2–13.

_____. 1969. The collie eye anomaly. JAVMA 155:859–65.

Roberts, S. R., and A. Dellaporta. 1965. Congenital posterior ectasia of the sclera in collie dogs. Part I. Clinical features. Am. J. Ophthalmol. 59:180–86.

Roberts, S. R., A. Dellaporta, and F. C. Winter. 1966. The collie ectasia syndrome: Pathology of eyes of pups one to fourteen days of age. Am. J. Ophthalmol. 61:1458–66.

_____. 1966. The collie ectasia syndrome: Pathology of the eyes of young and adult dogs. Am. J. Ophthalmol. 62:728–52.

Rubin, L. F. 1969. Collie eye anomaly: Comments. JAVMA 155:865–66.

Saunders, L. Z. 1952. Congenital optic nerve hypoplasia in collie dogs. Cornell Vet. 42:67–80.

Smythe, R. H. 1961. Hereditary defects in dogs. All Pets 32(9):15, 18.

_____. 1970. Hereditary defects. Vet. Rec. 86:240.

Sorsby, A., and J. B. Davey. 1954. Ocular associations of dappling (or merling) in the coat colour of dogs. I. Clinical and genetical data. J. Genet. 52:425–40.

Vainisi, S. J. 1969. Collie eye anomaly: Comments. JAVMA 155:876–77.

Whitehead, J. 1964. Hereditary defects of the ocular fundus in collies. NYC Vet. 7(6):7–9.

Wyman, M., and E. F. Donovan. 1969. Eye anomaly of the collie. JAVMA 155:866–70.

Yakely, W. L. 1972. Collie eye anomaly: Decreased prevalence through selective breeding. JAVMA 161:1103–7.

Yakely, W. L., M. Wyman, E. F. Donovan, and N. S. Fecheimer. 1968. Genetic transmission of an ocular fundus anomaly in collies. JAVMA 152:457–61.

Ectropion and Entropion

Ectropion, which may be acquired or congenital, refers to an eversion of the eyelid that results in the exposure of the conjunctival surface. Usually only the lower eyelid is affected.

Ectropion is common in the cocker spaniel, basset, mastiff, Great Dane, Saint Bernard, bloodhound, bulldog, boxer, English and Irish setters, and hound breeds. These are breeds with excessive skin on the lids and excessive length of palpebral fissure (eyelid slit). This causes the relaxation of the skin around the eyelids and the eyelids are pulled away from the globe. This leads to excessive drying, stagnation of tears in the lower fornix (angle between lower lid and eyeball), and in many cases eversion of the lacrimal punctum (lacrimal duct opening) so that lacrimal drainage is affected.

Infection of the conjunctiva is likely to occur, and the subsequent congestion may aggravate the malpositioning of the lid margin.

Overflow of tears is likely with the production of irritation of the skin of the lower lid.

Normal blinking is absent and this can lead to corneal problems.

Entropion is the inversion or turning inward of the eyelid. Subsequent irritation produced by the edge of the eyelid, the hair on the eyelid, or the eyelashes may lead to keratoconjunctivitis (inflammation of the external surface of the eye).

This condition has been observed in some 60 breeds of dogs but is most common in chow chows, cocker spaniels, golden retrievers, Labrador retrievers, bloodhounds, bull mastiffs, springer spaniels, Saint Bernards, bulldogs, Irish setters, papillons, Pomeranians, Norwegian elkhounds, poodles, and Irish wolfhounds. This condition may occur in conjunction with other defects. For example, in the cocker, entropion is often associated with ectropion in another part of the same lid. In the chow, entropion is usually associated with a small palpebral opening and a shortened lid. In the bloodhound and bull mastiff, the condition is associated with excessive folds of loose skin on the head.

Entropion is usually bilateral and may affect both the upper and lower lids. The lower lids are more commonly affected and the lateral margins are more commonly involved than the nasal border. Clinical signs include lacrimation (watery eyes), blepharospasm (blinking), conjunctival infection, photophobia (sensitivity to sunlight), epiphora (watery eyes due to failure of the tear duct, almost the same as lacrimation), prolapse of the nictitating membrane (third eyelid), pain, inflammation, keratitis, and ulceration.

The inversion of the eyelid causes the eye lashes, periorbital hair, and the edge of the eyelid to abrade or irritate the surface of the cornea and bulbar conjunctiva.

There is a continuous cycle of irritation. The entropion is responsible for the initial irritation and blepharospasm. Continued irritation initiates spasms of the orbicularis muscle so that not only the lashes but also the periorbital hair and tarsal plate (a fibrous plate in the eyelid) abrade. Entropion carries bacteria and dirt into the conjunctival sac. Keratitis (corneal inflammation) and eventual corneal ulceration and rupture may result from this continuous cycle.

INHERITANCE AND RECOMMENDATION. Limited observations, high incidence in certain breeds, and data based on other species suggest that entropion may be inherited as an autosomal dominant trait with complete penetrance. The specific mode of inheritance for ectropion is not reported in the literature.

Selection pressure against these traits should be stressed. Assuming a dominant mode of inheritance, the elimination of animals expressing this characteristic should reduce its incidence.

REFERENCES

Aguirre, G., Guest Editor. 1973. Vet. Clin. North Am.: Ophthalmol. Vol. 3, no. 3. Philadelphia, London, Toronto: W. B. Saunders.

Burns, M., and M. N. Fraser. 1966. The Genetics of the Dog. London: Oliver & Boyd, pp. 93–94.

Carter, J. D. 1972. Combined operation for noncicatrical entropion with distichiasis. JAAHA 8:53–58.

Dreyfus, M. 1953. Ectropion and entropion in dogs. Cesk. Ofthalmol. 9:57–58.

Halliwell, W. H. 1965. Undermined skin flaps as a method of entropion correction. Vet. Med. Small Anim. Clin. 60:915–19.

Hodgman, S. F. J. 1963. Abnormalities and defects in pedigree dogs. 1. An investigation into the existence of abnormalities in pedigree dogs in the Poretesh Isles. J. Small Anim. Pract. 4:447–56.

Koenig, C. W., and E. DePerro. 1970. Surgical correction of ectropion of the lower eyelid. (Report of a new technique.) Vet. Med. Small Anim. Clin. 65:243–46.

Menges, R. W. 1946. An operation for entropion in the dog. JAVMA 109:464–65.

Startup, F. G. 1960. Diseases of the canine eye. Vet. Rec. 72:653–60.

Wyman, M., E. F. Donovan, and R. L. Rudy. 1970. Surgical correction of cicatrical ectropion in the dog. Southwest Vet. 23:229–33.

Everted Membrana Nictitans (Third Eyelid)

An everted membrana nictitans refers to a condition that has been reported in certain large and medium-sized dogs such as the Great Dane, Weimaraner, Saint Bernard, Newfoundland, German shepherd, and German shorthaired pointer. The defect has been characterized by a unilateral or bilateral scroll-like curling forward of the cartilage of the membrane nictitans. Signs attributable to the anomaly are usually minimal and limited to epiphora (watery eyes) or a mucoid discharge.

PATHOPHYSIOLOGY. Histologic studies of the cartilage involved indicate normal cartilage.

INHERITANCE AND RECOMMENDATION. The mode of inheritance suggested for this defect based on limited data is a simple recessive.

Select against this defect as for any recessive until further evidence that a different type of gene action is involved.

REFERENCES

Gelatt, K. N. 1973. Pediatric ophthalmology in small animal practice. Vet. Clin. North Am.: Ophthalmol. 3(3):321–33. Philadelphia, London, Toronto: W. B. Saunders.
Martin, C. L., and R. Leach. 1970. Everted membrane nictitans in German shorthaired pointers. JAVMA 157:1229-32.

Glaucoma

Glaucoma refers to a group of ocular disorders that result in an increase in intraocular pressure. This increased pressure leads to structural damage and impairment of function. Glaucoma may result from an increased rate of aqueous humor production, but usually it is due to a narrowed iridocorneal angle, i.e., inadequate aqueous drainage. Glaucoma may be classified as primary, secondary, congenital, or absolute. Congenital glaucoma may also be classified as primary. Primary glaucoma refers to glaucoma in which the intraocular pressure increase is not the result of complications caused by previous ocular disease. Secondary glaucoma refers to an increase in intraocular pressure resulting from other known intraocular diseases or eye damage. Secondary glaucoma is more common than primary and is often unilateral, whereas primary glaucoma is usually bilateral, although both eyes need not be affected simultaneously. One eye may be affected before the other by a few days or up to 2 years. Congenital glaucoma results from a rise in intraocular pressure due to an eye malformation, such as an abnormality of the angle of the anterior chamber, which is present at birth. Absolute glaucoma or blindness is the final stage in any glaucoma. Two theories have been suggested as to the cause of primary glaucoma, and either of these or the combination of the two may be the cause. The first theory, neurovascular, suggests abnormal ocular circulation, which might occur on a local basis within the eye or as a consequence of a disturbance in the general circulation of the body as a whole. Contributing factors include disorders of the hypothalamic region, autonomic nervous system, or the endocrine system. The second, and perhaps more favored theory, is that it is mechanical. This refers to an actual blockage or inhibition of drainage. A common finding is an abnormal iridocorneal angle. The conversion of a narrow angle into one of complete closure is not well understood.

Primary glaucoma occurs for the most part in the American cocker spaniel but is also found in the basset hound. More recently it has been reported in beagles. In England, the condition has been reported in the miniature poodle, wirehaired terrier, poodle, Samoyed, English cocker, basset hound, and English springer spaniel. Primary glaucoma is a disease of older dogs, usually occurring between the ages of 3½ and 13 years.

Early clinical signs may go unnoticed by the dog's owner. The general clinical signs may include (not all in one individual) the following: increased intraocular pressure, pain, cloudy cornea, insensitive cornea, shallow anterior chamber, dilation of the pupil with no response to light, episcleral vascularization (congestion of the episcleral vessels), loss of vision (partial or complete), buphthalmos (hydrophthalmos), cupping of the optic disc, atrophy of the optic disc and retina, and atrophy of the iris. Acute glaucoma, at least in the cocker, appears to be somewhat seasonal and occurs most often from October to May.

PATHOPHYSIOLOGY. One observes an enlargement of the globe, a narrowed but not closed angle, atrophy of the ciliary body, choroid, and retina. Pannus (vascularization of the cornea) and congestion of the ciliary vessels may occur in an eye that has been subjected to numerous repeated attacks. Sagittal sections of the eye reveal the open angles of the anterior chamber and cupping in the optic disc.

An enlargement of the corneal epithelium reveals intracellular and intercellular edema. Atrophy and degeneration of the retina and the uveal tract nerve fiber occur, and the inner nuclear retinal layers are absent. Choroid is vascular with pigmentation. Lacunae in the optic nerve are visible in the cupped optic disc.

The aqueous humor in both chambers is formed and drained from the eye in the ciliary region; the ciliary processes are split with a ciliary cleft between them. The ciliary process consists of a central core of stroma and blood vessels covered by epithelium and is supplied by blood from the ciliary arteries. The aqueous humor is formed from all the blood vessels in the anterior part of the eye, but largely from the vessels within the ciliary processes. Diffusion and filtration of nonelectrolytes and electrolytes are involved in the formation of aqueous humor, with substances from the blood initiated by an enzymatic activity of the cells of the ciliary process. The aqueous humor is drained by way of a network of capillaries and veins forming an intrascleral plexus that is associated with the ciliary cleft and drains into the ciliary veins. The processes that make and remove the aqueous humor must be in balance to maintain normal intraocular pressure that is altered either by changes in the volume of aqueous humor within the eye or by some interference in outflow. Intraocular pressure may be greatly changed by differences in the rigidity of the sclera, by topical corticosteroids applied to the eye, an possibly by the myxedema of hypothyroidism.

INHERITANCE AND RECOMMENDATION. The definite mode of inheritance for glaucoma in the cocker spaniel has not been reported. The high incidence of this condition in the cocker, and perhaps the bassets, indicates a hereditary predisposition. A narrow iris angle in the cocker predisposes to acute congestive attacks. Glaucoma is reported to be inherited as a dominant or a recessive in humans. Limited data for the beagle suggest that glaucoma (with lens luxation) is inherited as an autosomal recessive trait.

Since the mode of inheritance is not well defined, specific recommendations cannot be made. The breeding of known affected animals and their close relatives should be discouraged. Elimination of this trait should be attempted in the same manner as for any other recessive or dominant genes.

REFERENCES

Barnett, D. C. 1970. Glaucoma in the dog. J. Small Anim. Pract. 11:113–28.
Bedford, P. G. C. 1975. The aetiology of primary glaucoma in the dog. J. Small Anim. Pract. 16:217–39.
Gelatt, K. N. 1972. Familial glaucoma in the beagle dog. JAAHA 8:23–28.
Lovekin, L. G. 1964. Primary glaucoma in dogs. JAVMA 145:1081–91.
Lovekin, L. G., and R. W. Bellhorn. 1968. Clinicopathologic changes in primary glaucoma in the cocker spaniel. Am. J. Vet. Res. 29:379–85.
Magrane, W. G. 1957. Canine glaucoma. I. Methods of diagnosis. JAVMA 131:311–14.
_____. 1957. Canine glaucoma. II. Primary classification. JAVMA 131:372–74.
_____. 1957. Canine glaucoma. IV. Medical and surgical treatment. JAVMA 131:456–64.
_____. 1971. Canine Ophthalmology. 2nd ed. Philadelphia: Lea & Febiger.
Martin, C. L., and M. Wyman. 1968. Glaucoma in the basset hound. JAVMA 153:1320–27.
Roberts, S. R. 1967. Recognizing glaucoma: The appearance, course, and effects of the disease in animal veterinary medicine. Proc. Am. Coll. Vet. Ophthalmol., Dallas, pp. 8–12.
Startup, F. G. 1969. Diseases of the canine eye. Baltimore: Williams & Wilkins.

Hemeralopia (Day Blindness)

An inherited condition exists in the Alaskan malamute in which the dogs are capable of seeing in decreased light (night) but cannot see in bright light (daylight). A similar condition may exist in the miniature poodle. The condition is usually first observed when the pup reaches 6–10 weeks of age.

PATHOPHYSIOLOGY. Dogs have normal direct and consensual pupillary reflexes, normal appearance of the retina, and absence of nystagmus.

INHERITANCE AND RECOMMENDATION. The mode of inheritance for day blindness is apparently autosomal recessive.

Select against this gene as for any recessive. Apparently selection has been effective.

REFERENCES

Aguirre, G. 1973. Hereditary retinal disease in small animals. Vet. Clin. North Am. 3:515–28.
Rubin, L. F., T. K. R. Bourns, and L. H. Lord. 1967. Hemeralopia in dogs: Hereditary hemeralopia in Alaskan malamute. Am. J. Vet. Res. 28:355–57.

Lens Luxation

Luxation (dislocation) of the crystalline lens implies that the lens is not found in its normal location but is lying either in the anterior chamber in front of the iris or behind the iris not within the hyaloid fossa. This condition may be congenital or acquired. Acquired luxation of the lens is usually the result of an injury.

Luxation occurs due to the complete disruption of the ligamentous attachment. Luxation of the crystalline lens is a heritable defect in certain breeds of dogs. This condition is confined for the most part to wirehaired and smooth fox terriers, Jack Russell terriers, and the Sealyham terriers. Cases have been reported in Webster terriers, greyhounds, German shepherds, corgis, miniature poodles, French bulldogs, Labrador retrievers, border collies, and Scottish terriers. Luxation is usually bilateral, but the condition in one eye may precede that of the other. The lens may subluxate or dislocate, usually into the anterior chamber. If the luxation of the lens is into the anterior chamber, secondary glaucoma may follow and lead to gross damage to the eye.

Clinical signs usually appear between 3 and 7 years of age. The onset of lens displacement produces a considerable variation in clinical signs. It has been reported that blindness may occur overnight, with the owner of the dog reporting excessive barking by the dog. Reduced vision may be observed several days before the lens are free. Blepharospasm and lacrimation may be observed. One may observe dilation of the pupil, the eye partly closed, and the dog rubbing the eye. The dog may lie in a dark area and avoid exposure to light.

Iridodenesis or trembling of the iris may be observed with the movement of the dog's head or eyes.

PATHOPHYSIOLOGY. The dislocation of the lens is actually due to rupture of the suspensory ligament. This leaves the lens without support and leads to iridodenesis and to anterior uveitis (inflammation of the iris), resulting in an increase in the protein content of aqueous humor. There is consequent interference with filtration of the fluid, a rise in intraocular tension, and secondary glaucoma.

Buphthalmos (enlarged eye) from glaucoma may result in acquired secondary lens luxation.

INHERITANCE AND RECOMMENDATION. No detailed studies have been conducted on the mode of inheritance of lens luxation (defective zonule). The high incidence in certain breeds strongly suggests an inherited defect at least for those breeds.

Since the exact mode of inheritance is not well documented, it would be suggested that affected animals not be used for breeding and that close relatives of affected animals be carefully observed.

REFERENCES

Albert, R. A. 1973. Luxation of the canine lens. Auburn Vet. 128:99–103.

Chandler, F. A. 1970. Lens luxation in the Webster terrier. Vet. Rec. 86:145–46.

Formston, C. 1945. Observations on subluxation and luxation of the crystalline lens in the dog. J. Comp. Pathol. 55:168–84.

_____. 1952. Observations on diseases of the eye in animals with particular reference to the dog. Vet. Rec. 64:47–49.

Gelatt, K. N. 1971. Glaucoma and lens luxation in a dog. Vet. Med. Small Anim. Clin. 66:1102–4.

Lawson, D. D. 1969. Luxation of the crystalline lens in the dog. J. Small Anim. Pract. 10:461–63.

_____. 1970. Luxation of the crystalline lens in the dog. Trans. Ophthalmol. Soc. U.K. 89:259–62.

Magrane, W. G. 1957. Canine glaucoma. III. Secondary classification. JAVMA 131:374–78.

_____. 1971. Canine Ophthalmology. 2nd ed. Philadelphia: Lea & Febiger.

Wright, J. G. 1937. Clinical case records, Beaumont Hospital, Royal Veterinary College.

Microphthalmia (with Colobomas)

Hereditary microphthalmia with colobomas (defects) refers to an inherited congenital eye defect found in the Australian shepherd. Similar ocular anomalies have been reported in Shetland sheepdogs from merle-to-merle matings. This defect appears to be associated with coat color and to be related to excessive white coats (30%–90% white) and lack of merling. However, excessive white-blue merle Australian shepherds have been found free from the defect. The anomalies occur in both sexes and generally in both eyes, although the condition may be asymmetric.

PATHOPHYSIOLOGY. All the affected dogs expressed microphthalmia, microcornea, and iridal heterochromia with dyscoria (pupil abnormal shaped) and corectopia (pupil off center). Over 50% of the dogs had cataracts, equatorial staphylomas, and retinal detachment.

The fundus pattern was subalbinotic type. There was an absence of tapetum lucidum (reflective layer of the eye) and only slight pigmentation of the nontapetal fundus.

INHERITANCE AND RECOMMENDATION. The data presented suggest that this trait may be inherited as an autosomal recessive.

Select against this trait as one would any recessive gene. Consider, however, that the merle gene is dominant and that as suggested for the sheltie, a double merle mating results in the possible white pup, expressing the condition. Merle-to-merle mating is not recommended.

REFERENCES

Aguirre, G. 1973. Hereditary retinal disease in small animals. Vet. Clin. North Am. 3:515–28.

Gelatt, K. N., and L. D. McGill. 1970. Clinical characteristics of microphthalmia with colobomas. Vet. Med. Small Anim. Clin. 65:39–42.

Persistent Pupillary Membrane

Persistent pupillary membrane is a congenital eye defect observed frequently (some suggest incidence of 40%) in the basenji and occasionally in other breeds. This condition may be associated with other ocular defects but may also occur as an isolated anomaly. The expression of this defect may vary between individuals from those that are not visually handicapped with lesions difficult to distinguish to those with gross lesions of the cornea, iris, or lens and affected vision.

Normally, atrophy of the pupillary membrane begins during fetal life and is complete by the time the pup is 3–8 weeks of age. In the basenji, atrophy may proceed at a slower pace (2 weeks to 8 months). If a portion of the pupillary membrane does not atrophy and remains into adult life, it is referred to as a persistent pupillary membrane.

One or both eyes may be affected. Usually the condition is bilateral but not necessarily symmetrical.

PATHOPHYSIOLOGY. The pupillary membrane has been described as a sheet of mesoderm carrying a network of anastomosing blood vessels, covering the anterior surface of the lens, and formed during the embryonic development of the eye. It forms a very thin and almost acellular central part of the lamina iridopupillaris, or posterior wall of the anterior chamber, the peripheral portion of which remains permanently to form the superficial layer of the iris.

Atrophy of the pupillary membrane usually occurs at 2–3 weeks of age, beginning at the center of the pupil and leaving a few strands visible around the edge, finally disappearing by 3–8 weeks of age. Atrophy normally proceeds somewhat slower in the basenji, i.e., from 2 weeks later to a few months in some cases.

Two theories have been set forth as to cause. The first is that the pupillary membrane and all the anterior segment defects attributed to them are the result of faulty mesodermal development with possible aberrant differentiation of the corneal tissue. The second theory is that all forms of persistent pupillary membranes and associated anomalies in the eye of the basenji are the result of the presence of typical colobomas.

Anomalies associated with persistent pupillary membrane include:

(1) Prominent minor vascular circle (iris collarette 3–5 times as thick as normal) in which portions of the iris vessel project into the anterior chamber. Spaces are formed between the vessel and iris surface colobomation in the form of small circular holes in the border of the iris.

(2) Corneal opacities: (a) Localized corneal opacity with discrete white dots or linear or branching opacities localized in the region of Descement's membrane (innermost layer of the cornea). (b) Diffuse small or large opacities of the deep corneal layers. Multiple, pleomorphic (varying in

shape), gray or white lesions with indistinct borders affecting the central or paracentral portion of the cornea. (c) Corneal stromae adjacent to lesions. Descement's membrane appears more granular than normal. Pigmented bands of the pupillary membrane stretch from the inner aspect of the cornea at the site of the corneal opacities to the iris face, where they attach at the region of the minor vascular circle.

(3)   Anterior polar cataract. An eye with this lesion has small or large, single or multiple, discrete or diffuse opacities occupying the central or paracentral portion of the pupil. Most are confined to the surface of the anterior lens capsule.

Various forms of colobomata of the disc have also been reported.

INHERITANCE AND RECOMMENDATION. The literature is not in agreement as to the exact mode of inheritance for persistent pupillary membrane. It has been suggested by one group of investigators that, if the wide variations in expression are all classed as typical colobomata and are considered together from a genetic standpoint, this condition follows a dominant genetic pattern with no sex linkage. The gene apparently varies in expression and penetrance. Other workers have stated that this condition is not subject to a simple dominant or simple recessive form of inheritance. They stated, however, that there is a variation in expressivity and incomplete penetrance.

If dominant, the removal of dogs with the condition would eliminate the trait from the kennel. If recessive, a breeding test would be needed. A breeding test might also be required when penetrance is incomplete.

Progressive Retinal Atrophy

Progressive retinal atrophy is characterized by a progressive bilateral symmetrical degeneration of the visual elements of the retina. Two types or forms of progressive retinal atrophy have been reported. The first type, generalized progressive retinal atrophy (PRA) or peripheral, is due to a simple autosomal recessive gene. The second type, central progressive retinal atrophy (CPRA), probably results from a dominant gene, with incomplete penetrance (penetrance 80%); however, in some breeds CPRA may be due to a recessive gene, or it is possible that both dominant and recessive genes may influence this trait in the same breed. Both types are progressive and cause blindness. With PRA, night vision is gradually lost and day vision remains normal. In the next stage the dog has complete night blindness, with day vision deteriorating. In the third stage the animal is completely blind and secondary cataracts often develop in some breeds. Also an early loss of peripheral vision may be noted, with resulting "tunnel vision"; i.e., the dog sees only objects directly in front of it.

With CPRA, night blindness is not frequently observed. Dogs may be able to see better in dull light than in bright light. Dogs with CPRA have poor near vision and have difficulty in seeing still objects but can see moving objects until the latter stages of the disease. Peripheral vision may be retained for some time. Blind spots in the dogs' vision may occur.

Degeneration begins in the first few weeks of the pups' lives, and loss of vision is progressive, with complete loss of vision occurring in early to mid adulthood, dependent somewhat on breed. Progressive retinal atrophy has been identified in at least 46 breeds, for example, Irish setters, miniature and toy poodles, cocker spaniels, miniature pinschers, Labrador retrievers, golden retrievers, huskies, Norwegian elkhounds, Samoyeds, English cockers, collies, Akitas, and salukis. CPRA is common in Labrador retrievers, border collies, English springer spaniels, golden retrievers, and Shetland sheepdogs. Careful selection and good breeding practices have been extremely successful in reducing its frequency. Breed differences are noted as to time of development and electrophysiology.

Eye examination, when PRA is present, reveals a dilated pupil with poor and slow pupillary light reflex, although some reflex is retained even in advanced cases. When present, a cataract follows the course of the retinal atrophy, beginning as a cortical cataract both posterior and anterior, and ending as a total cataract.

Examination of the fundus shows the most obvious signs of narrowing of the retinal blood vessels, both arteries and veins. This sign is most easily seen in the vessels crossing the tapetum, the venous circle on the disc remaining until the end. There is pallor of the optic disc and increased reflection from the tapetal region, which becomes silvery and mirrorlike in its appearance. The tapetum nigrum becomes pale gray, sometimes with darker pigment scattered about. With CPRA, the pupil is dilated, but not in the early stages, and there is less associated cataract. The retinal changes start at the area centralis or macular region, soon spreading to the rest of the tapetal region and therefore involving the central retina. The first change is an increased reflection and pigmentary disturbance, small clouds and irregular spots of brown pigment appearing scattered over the tapetum lucidum and between these pigment spots the surface is highly reflective. The tapetum nigrum is not affected until much later, and whether the whole retina becomes finally affected is debatable, some normal peripheral retina remaining for a long time. Attenuation of the retinal vessels also occurs but late in the course of the disease.

PHYSIOPATHOLOGY. Histologic studies, at least for some breeds, indicate that following birth the retina develops normally for 18–21 days, after which spontaneous degeneration of the rods begins, until the final stage of degeneration occurs with complete disorganization of the retinal layers.

In stage 1 of PRA, one observes atrophy of rods and their nuclei. In stage 2, final disintegration of the cones occurs and the external limiting membrane now lies against the pigment epithelium. In stage 3, the outer nuclear layer is reduced to a layer of cone nuclei. The inner nuclear layer is almost normal, as well as the ganglion cells. Pigmented epithelium is devoid of pigment even in the nontapetal fundus. Choriocapillaries are much reduced. Later in this stage the changes proceeded to sclerosis. An irregular single nuclear layer is formed and the whole retina is greatly reduced in thickness. Later still, there is a definite thinning of the choroid with a reduction of its blood vessels. Different pathologic processes occur in different breeds. For example, rod dysplasia in the elkhound, progressive rod-cone degeneration in the miniature poodles, rod-cone dysplasia in the Irish setter, and cone degeneration in the malamute.

The histopathologic changes of CPRA are hypertrophy and migration of the pigment epithelium cells and loss of the layer of rods and cones. The large pigment-laden cells migrate through the retina and form cell nests on its inner surface. By this time the retina is disorganized. The changes occur in the central region and there is a sharp division between the affected and the unaffected peripheral retina.

INHERITANCE. Indications are, as previously mentioned, that generalized progressive retinal atrophy is inherited as a simple autosomal recessive gene (toy and miniature poodles, Norwegian elkhound, Irish setter, Alaskan malamute). Central progressive retinal atrophy is inherited as a dominant in some breeds (Labrador), but in at least one breed, a dominant as well as a recessive mode of inheritance may be involved.

RECOMMENDATION. For PRA (recessive), any individual animals exhibiting this trait should not be used for breeding. A breeding test could be established to detect carrier individuals. Selection has been extremely successful in Irish setters. Test mating is less practical in breeds where the defect develops later in life.

For CPRA, do not use the dog expressing this trait for breeding.

Apparently there is no treatment for the condition.

REFERENCES

Aguirre, G. D., and L. F. Rubin. 1971. Progressive retinal atrophy (rod dysplasia) in the Norwegian elkhound. JAVMA 158:208–18.

———. 1971. The early diagnosis of rod dysplasia in the Norwegian elkhound. JAVMA 159:429–33.

———. 1972. Progressive retinal atrophy in the miniature poodle: An electrophysiologic study. JAVMA 160:191–201.

———. 1975. Rod-cone dysplasia (progressive retinal atrophy) in Irish setters. JAVMA 166:157–64.

Barnett, K. C. 1962. Hereditary retinal atrophy in the poodle. Vet. Rec. 74:672–75.

———. 1965. Canine retinopathies. I. History and review of the literature. J. Small Anim. Pract. 6:41–45.

_____. 1965. Canine retinopathies. II. The miniature and toy poodle. J. Small Anim. Pract. 6:93–109.

_____. 1965. Two forms of hereditary and progressive retinal atrophy in the dog. I. The miniature poodle. II. The Labrador retriever. Anim. Hosp. 1:234–45.

_____. 1969. Genetic anomalies of the posterior segments of the canine eye. J. Small Anim. Pract. 10:451–55.

_____. 1969. Primary retinal dystrophies in the dog. JAVMA 154:804–8.

Barnett, K. C., and W. L. Dunn. 1969. The International Sheep Dog Society and progressive retinal atrophy. J. Small Anim. Pract. 10:301–7.

Black, L. 1969. The progressive retinal atrophy scheme. Vet. Rec. 85:694–95.

_____. 1972. Progressive retinal atrophy: A review of the genetics and an appraisal of the eradication scheme. J. Small Anim. Pract. 13:295–314.

Cogan, D. G., and T. Kuwabara. 1965. Photoreceptive abiotrophy of the retina in the elkhound. Pathol. Vet. 2:101–28.

Gelatt, K. N. 1974. Description and diagnosis of progressive retinal atrophy. Norden News (Spring), pp. 24–34.

Hodgman, S. F. J., H. B. Parry, W. J. Rasbridge, and J. D. Steel. 1949. Progressive retinal atrophy in dogs. I. The disease in Irish setters (red). Vet. Rec. 61:185–89.

Keep, J. M. 1972. Clinical aspects of progressive retinal atrophy in the Carigan Welsh corgi. Aust. Vet. J. 48:197–99.

Kirk, R. W. 1971. Current Veterinary Therapy. Philadelphia: W. B. Saunders.

Parry, H. B. 1953. Degeneration of the dog retina. II. Generalized progressive atrophy of hereditary origin. Br. J. Ophthalmol. 37:487–502.

Patterson, D. G., and W. Medway. 1966. Hereditary diseases of the dog. JAVMA 149:1741–54.

Peiffer, R. L., and K. N. Gelatt. 1975. Progressive retinal atrophy in two atypical breeds of dogs. Vet. Med. Small Anim. Clin. 70:1476–78.

Priester, W. A. 1974. Canine progressive retinal atrophy: Occurrence by age, breed, and sex. Am. J. Vet. Res. 35(4):571–74.

Startup, F. G. 1969. Diseases of the canine eye. Baltimore: Williams & Wilkins.

von Krahenmann, A. 1974. Progressive netzhautatrophie bei schweizer hunderassen. 1. Mitterlung: periphere netzhautatrophie. Schweiz. Arch. Tierheilkd. 116:643–52.

Retinal Dysplasia

Retinal dysplasia (improper development of the retina) is an inherited bilateral defect causing total blindness due to a detached retina and is found most often in Bedlington terriers, Sealyham terriers, and Labrador retrievers. Detachment is usually complete and conical and is present within a completely liquified vitrous body. As the animal gets older, the frequency of vitrous hemorrhage increases. Both sexes are affected. The condition may be present at birth but is usually first noticed in the pup at approximately 3–8 weeks of age. Clinically affected pups have a vacant expression, are less adventurous, less lively, and are clumsy. Such pups will be blind.

PATHOPHYSIOLOGY. The dog has a detached retina and in some cases some degree of microphthalmos. There may be a pupillary light reflex and frequently a rapid and intermittent nystagmus. The retinal attachment to the ora serrata is incomplete or consists in some places of a thin transparent sheet.

In the newborn pup the retina appears edematous, folded, and in some cases has a defect between the retina and ora serrata. At first small folds appear near the papilla in an otherwise normal retina. Changes also include edema in the inner nuclear layer of the retina, which in places divides the retina into large and small cysts. There is formation of rosettes with a marked basal membrane and later degeneration of the rods and cones, and peripherally next to the ora serrata there is a thin sheet of cells connected to the detached retina. In some cases the free end of the detached and disenserted retina can be seen.

The lens show different grades of posterior cortical cataract.

INHERITANCE AND RECOMMENDATION. The trait appears to result from a recessive gene with complete penetrance.

Select against this gene as for any recessive gene.

REFERENCES

Aguirre, G. 1973. Hereditary retinal disease in small animals. Vet. Clin. North Am. 3:515–28.

Ashton, N., K. C. Barnett, and D. D. Sachs. 1968. Retinal dysplasia in the Sealyham terrier. J. Pathol. 96:269–72.

Barnett, K. C. 1969. Genetic anomalies of the posterior segment of the canine eye. J. Small Anim. Pract. 10:451–55.

Barnett, K. C., G. R. Bjorch, and E. Kock. 1970. Hereditary retinal dysplasia in the Labrador retriever in England and Sweden. J. Small Anim. Pract. 10:755–59.

Rubin, L. F. 1963. Hereditary retinal detachment in Bedlington terriers: A preliminary report. Small Anim. Clin. 3:387–89.

___, 1968. Heredity of retinal dysplasia in Bedlington terriers. JAVMA 152:260–62.

Trichiasis and Distichia

Trichiasis refers to eyelashes that arise from their normal position but their direction or angle of growth is abnormal so they impinge on either the conjunctiva or cornea. This condition is found in many breeds such as the poodle, Pekingese, boxer, collie, pug, dachshund, Shetland sheepdog, bulldog, fox terrier, and Chihuahua. Abrasion of the cornea by the eyelashes produces excessive lacrimation and irritation, which may lead to conjunctivitis or keratitis and eventually to superficial corneal vascularization or ulceration.

Distichia is a congenital anomaly that results in two rows of eyelashes along the margin of the eyelid instead of one. The second row erupts from the position of the Meibomian glands along the posterior border of the eyelid. These rows may be partial or complete. The number of abnormal lashes varies from 1 to 20. The lashes from the inner row curve inward and impinge on the cornea leading to conjunctivitis and keratitis. Either or both lids (usually the upper) may be affected and the extra lashes are usually nonpigmented. The condition is common in cocker spaniels, Pekingese, and poodles, but does occur in other breeds such as Bedlington terriers, pugs, dachshunds, boxers, German shepherds, chows, wirehaired fox terriers, English bulldogs, Boston terriers, English and Irish setters, Saint Bernards, Shetland sheepdogs, collies, springer spaniels, Chihuahuas, Pomeranians, and retrievers. Clinical signs include epiphora, irritation, photophobia, and hyperemia of the conjunctiva.

The primary defect is related to the Meibomian glands. The typical canine lid has 20–25 Meibomian glands along the lid margin. The glands may be smaller than normal, absent, or replaced by atavistic (characteristic of earlier biological types) sebaceous glands. The result is that a second row of small, usually nonpigmented cilia erupt and curve or grow inward and irritate the eye. The condition may be observed accompanying ectropion due to a lack of support by the rudimentary tarsal plate of the eyelid, diminution of the palpebral fissure by itself or in conjunction with microphthalmia, and the absence of one or both lacrimal punctums and canaliculi.

Cilia abrade the globe of the eye producing conjunctivitis, photophobia, epiphora, and eventual corneal ulceration and perforation. A variation has been reported where the eyelashes emerge through the tarsal conjunctiva. This occurred in the Doberman, Pekingese, miniature schnauzer, and Shih Tzu.

INHERITANCE AND RECOMMENDATION. Canine distichia is reported in the literature to be due to an autosomal dominant gene with incomplete penetrance. However, this needs much further study. The specific pattern of inheritance of trichiasis is not reported in the literature.

Breeders should select against dogs showing these traits. Removal of the dogs exhibiting these traits should reduce their incidence.

REFERENCES

Bedford, P. G. 1973. Distichiasis and its treatment by the method of partial tarsal plate excision. J. Small Anim. Pract. 14:1–5.

Bellhorn, R. W. 1970. Variations of canine distichiasis. JAVMA 157:342–43.

Carter, J. D. 1972. Combined operation for noncicatrical entropion with distichiasis. JAAHA 8(1):53–58.

Gelatt, K. N. 1969. Resection of cilia-bearing tarsoconjunctiva for correction of canine distichia. JAVMA 155:892–97.

_____. 1971. Bilateral corneal dermoids and distichiasis in a dog. Vet. Med. Small Anim. Clin. 66:658–59.

Halliwell, W. H. 1967. Surgical management of canine distichia. JAVMA 150:874–79.

Helper, L. C., and W. G. Magrane. 1970. Ectopic cilia of the canine eyelid. J. Small Anim. Pract. 11:185–89.

Hodgman, S. F. J. 1962. Abnormalities of possible hereditary origin in dogs. Vet. Rec. 74:1239–46.

Panel Report, Part I. 1972. Distichiasis. Mod. Vet. Pract. 53(6):65–67.

Panel Report, Part II. 1972. Distichiasis. Mod. Vet. Pract. 53(7):55–57.

Startup, F. G. 1969. Diseases of the canine eye. Baltimore: Williams & Wilkins.

EAR (DEAFNESS)

Deafness, like any other defect, may be congenital or acquired. All cases of congenital deafness are not inherited. Deafness may occur in any breed but is much more common in certain breeds, and for these breeds it is believed to be inherited. Examples are the Dalmatian, bull terrier, Sealyham, Scotch terrier, border collie, fox terrier, foxhound, Great Dane, collie, Shetland sheepdog, dachshund, Norwegian dunkerhound, poodle, and Rottweiler.

Deafness in some breeds appears to be linked to coat color, i.e., in bull terriers, Sealyhams, and Dalmatians—those with a lack of pigment, such as white dogs or dogs with a predominance of white markings. In some breeds dominant spotting when homozygous produces the defect along with blindness and general weakness in pups (dappled dachshund, merled sheltie or collie, Harlequin Dane). The heterozygote is frequently "walleyed" with the tapetum rudimentary or lacking.

Pathophysiology

The pathology of deafness expressed by the various breeds no doubt differs. For the foxhound it was found that a bulbous growth (myxoma) enveloped the stapes (middle ear) and functionally separated the stapes from the oval window. What appeared to be new bone formation was found in the area where the cochlea normally lies. The organ of Corti, scala tympani, and scala vestibule (parts of the inner ear) were absent and the area contained tissue similar to skin.

In the Dalmatian, spotting is recessive and the spots do not have white hair. Therefore, a different pattern of defects (lesions) could be expected. The lesions for the Dalmatian have been summarized as follows: in the young dog there is collapse of the cochlear duct, degeneration of the hair cells of the organ of Corti, and collapse of the saccule. Some reports also include degeneration of the spiral ganglion cells, the acoustic nerve, and various segments of the central auditory system. Age difference in dogs studied could well account for these differences.

For the collie, the tectorial membrane appeared to have solidified and is made up of a coagulum. In cross sections it has the appearance of a shelf projecting into the scala media (cochlear duct) cells lying on top of the tectorial membrane. The cells appeared to be the remains of degenerated pillar and hair cells. This peculiar tectorial membrane was not found throughout the chochlea but mainly in the upper half of the second turn.

Inheritance

For the Dalmatian with the degenerative type of deafness, a recessive mode of inheritance is suggested, but additional proof is still needed if recessive penetrance is not complete. More recent evidence suggests a sex-linked gene with incomplete penetrance in the female heterozygote. The gene must also vary in expressivity since varying degrees of deafness are noted.

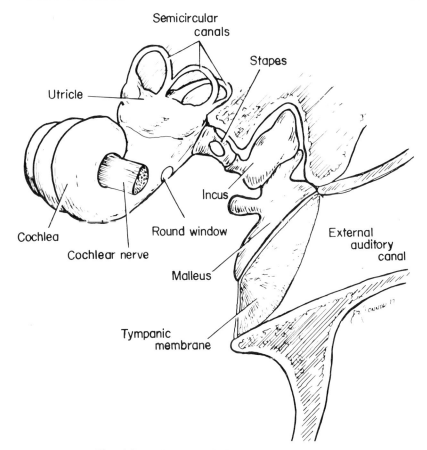

Fig. 4.2. *Diagram of the auditory apparatus. Sound waves are transmitted from the auditory canal via three bones (malleus, incus, stapes) to the cochlea, and impulses generated there are transmitted to the brain via the cochlear nerve for interpretation. The semicircular canals lie in three planes and keep the animal aware of its spatial orientation.*

For the breeds in which the double merle gene is involved, the double merle (homozygous merle) results in the complete expression of the trait.

Recommendation

Avoid the mating of two merles (or Harlequins). This will prevent the defect from being fully expressed.

For Dalmatians, select against the defect, considering it as both a sex-linked and/or recessive condition.

REFERENCES

Adams, E. W. 1956. Hereditary deafness in a family of foxhounds. JAVMA 128:302-3.

Anderson, H., B. Henricson, P. G. Lundquist, E. Wedenberg, and J. Wersall. 1968. Genetic hearing impairment in the Dalmatian dog. Acta Oto-Laryngol. Suppl. 232, pp. 1-34.

Catcott, E. J., and J. F. Smithcors (eds.). 1973. Prog. Canine Pract. 2(3):563.

Fraser, J. S. 1924. Congenital deafness in a white bull terrier puppy. J. Laryngol. Otol. 39:92-95.

Hodgman, S. F. J. 1962. Abnormalities of possible hereditary origin in dogs. Vet. Rec. 74:1239-46.

Hudson, W. R., N. C. Durham, and R. J. Ruben. 1962. Hereditary deafness in the Dalmatian dog. Arch. Otolaryngol. 75:213-19.

Lurie, M. H. 1948. The membranous labyrinth in the congenitally deaf collie and Dalmatian dog. Laryngoscope 58:279-87.

Phillips, J. McI., and E. D. Knight. 1938. Merle or calico foxhounds. J. Hered. 29:365-67.

Sorsby, A., and J. B. Davey. 1954. Ocular associations of dappling (or merling) in the coat color of dogs. I. Clinical and genetical data. J. Genet. 52:425-40.

Winge, O. 1950. Inheritance in Dogs with Special Reference to Hunting Breeds. Ithaca, N.Y.: Comstock Publ. Co.

Young, G. B. 1955. Inherited defects in dogs. Vet. Rec. 67:15-19.

CHAPTER 5

Bones and Joints

ACHONDROPLASIA

Achondroplasia or chondrodystrophy is the failure of the cartilage to develop properly—the deficient growth of bones derived from a cartilage matrix. It is difficult for dog breeders to agree on what is normal, but if one accepts as normal the structure of the so-called wild type or original ancestor of the dog, several breeds exhibit pronounced achondroplasia of either the limbs or axial skeleton or both. These breeds are characterized by localized deformities.

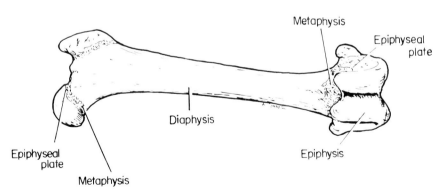

Fig. 5.1. *Structure of a long bone. Growth in length occurs at the epiphyseal plate and into the metaphysis. Developmental defects commonly cause malformation in the epiphyseal-metaphyseal area.*

Extremities

Shortness of leg in the dog is due to a dominant gene. This is true of the breeds with short, straight legs and also of the dogs with short, twisted, and distorted legs (achondroplasia).

The epiphyseal growth cartilages in the extremities fail to give the usual longitudinal proliferation of cartilage cells as forerunners for the normal growth in length of long bones, but instead, the cartilage is abnormally scant and the cellular proliferation and growth take place in transverse spirals and other irregular directions.

The trait is dominant in breeds tested. The expression of the trait varies in severity due to other bone characteristics (type and length of bone) of the breeds concerned. Also, when heterozygous, an intermediate degree of phenotypic expression (closer to the short-limbed parent, but nevertheless distinguishable) may be observed in some crosses.

REFERENCES

Braund, K. G., P. Ghosh, T. K. F. Taylor, and L. H. Larsen. 1975. Morphological studies of the canine intervertebral disc: The assignment of the beagle to the achondroplastic classification. Rec. Vet. Sci. 19:167–72.

Gardner, D. L. 1959. Familial canine chondrodystrophia factalis (achondroplasia). J. Pathol. Bacteriol. 77:243–47.

Ghosh, P., T. K. F. Taylor, K. G. Braund, and L. H. Larson. 1975. Genetic factors in the maturation of the canine intervertebral disc. Rec. Vet. Sci. 19:304–11.

Hansen, H. J. 1952. A pathologic-anatomical study in disc degeneration in the dog. Acta Orthop. Scand. Suppl. 11:1–117.

Hoerlein, B. F. 1971. Canine Neurology: Diagnosis and Treatment, p. 321. 2nd ed. Philadelphia, London, Toronto: W. B. Saunders.

Russell, S. W., and R. C. Griffiths. 1968. Recurrence of cervical disc syndrome in surgically and conservatively treated dogs. JAVMA 153:1412–31.

Stockard, C. R. 1941. The genetic and endocrine basis for differences in form and behavior. Philadelphia: Wistar Institute of Anatomy and Biology.

Axial Skeleton, Skull, and Vertebral Column

The inheritance of skull modifications is complex. The modifications of the different parts or structures of the skull are inherited more or less independently of each other, and because of this, frequent disharmonies are observed among the parts resulting in functional inefficiency. Both dominant and recessive inheritance are involved. For example, factors with the shorter upper face and jaw are not closely associated with those that influence the length of the lower jaw. (A complex of both dominant and recessive factors are involved.)

Length of tail and bent tail (screw tail) may involve two pairs of recessive genes—one pair for short tail and one pair for bent tail. In combination with the homozygous alleles for short tail, straight is not fully dominant over bent, but it is completely dominant over bent tails in the long tail. The fusion and shortening of caudal vertebrae resulting in a decrease in tail length are inherited independently from the vertebrae deformity that produces bending or twisting. Here, as with limbs, a defect is noted in the growth of cartilage and bone but is localized in the skull and caudal end of the vertebral column.

Achondroplasia (chondrodystrophia foetalis) has been found in breeds where it is not usually expected. This condition can be observed in the young pup prior to weaning. The pup stands with difficulty and is unable to walk without falling forward. In these pups the appendicular skeleton is abnormal. The enlarged ends of the long bone are cartilaginous in nature and the excess cartilage causes an apparent increase in the joint spaces. The calcified ends of the diaphyses (shaft of the bone) are splayed out with pointed margins at the periosteal bodies. The epiphyseal centers of ossification are located unusually near the diaphyses and are small and occasionally cradled in Y-shaped bone ends. All long bones are affected. Costochondral junctions are large and prominent. The vertebral column has a mild dorsal kyphosis (hump), and the vertebral bodies are small and misshapen. The skull is normal. Calcification appears normal.

INHERITANCE AND RECOMMENDATION. This condition in the miniature poodle, based on one report, appears as a simple recessive.

Select against this trait as for any recessive.

REFERENCES

Gardner, D. L. 1959. Familial canine chondrodystrophia foetalis (achondroplasia). J. Pathol. Bacteriol. 77:243–47.
Stockard, C. R. 1941. The genetic and endocrine basis for differences in form and behavior. Philadelphia: Wistar Institute of Anatomy and Biology.

Anury (Tailess)

Congenital anury has been reported in the cocker. Apparently this condition is very rare. The condition varied in expression from no tail in one kennel to at least one pup in a second kennel with one caudal vertebra.

Tailessness in the families of cockers probably resulted from a recessive gene. This condition, if present, could be eliminated by using selection against a recessive gene.

REFERENCE

Pullig, T. 1953. Anury in cocker spaniels. J. Hered. 44:105–7.

BRACHYURY

Dogs born with short tails in breeds that normally have long tails have been reported—for example, cocker spaniel, beagle, and toy griffon. Often one notices a considerable degree of distortion in the short tail. This could also be a variation of the gene for absence of tail.

Inheritance and Recommendation

The type of inheritance for short tail seems to vary between breeds. In the toy griffon the short tail was dominant to the long tail. In the cocker the short tail was probably recessive. In a colony of beagles selected for short tails, the gene was considered to be an autosomal dominant with reduced penetrance. Variation in segmental locus and type of skeletal abnormality is apparently multifactorial since selective breeding for shorter tails reduces the number of caudal vertebrae in successive generations. In crosses between the basset (long tail) and the bulldog, the pups had long, straight tails. Back crosses suggested that two pairs of genes were involved. One for long-short tail and one for straight-kinky tail. Long is dominant to short and straight dominant to kinky.

Elimination of these traits would vary according to breed and type of inheritance. Dogs with dominant traits may be removed following observation, and dogs with recessive traits should be eliminated following breeding tests.

REFERENCES

Curtis, R. D., D. English, and Y. J. Kim. 1964. Spina bifida in a "stub" dog stock, selectively bred for short tails. Anat. Rec. 148:365.
Little, C. C. 1934. Inheritance in toy griffons. J. Hered. 25:198–201.
Pullig, T. 1957. Brachyury in cocker spaniels. J. Hered. 48:75–76.
Stockard, C. R., et al. 1941. The genetic and endocrine basis for differences in form and behavior. Philadelphia: Wistar Institute of Anatomy and Biology.

CARPAL SUBLUXATION

A sex-linked recessive trait, carpal dislocation, has been reported in a group of experimental dogs. Pups appear normal at birth, and a gradual change begins at about 3 weeks of age when the pups first attempt to walk. The final degree of adult dislocation is varied.

The limb deformity is limited to the carporadial joints and always occurs bilaterally. No primary anatomical or physiologic basis has been discovered for this condition.

Inheritance and Recommendation

Subluxation of the carpal joints of both front limbs is a sex-linked recessive trait (X chromosome) closely linked with the locus for canine hemophilia A. However, pups affected with both subluxation and hemophilia A. However, pups affected with both subluxation and hemophilia have not been observed, suggesting the genes are in repulsion in the double heterozygote, and crossing-over has not occurred.

See previously listed technique for a sex-linked trait as outlined under hemophilia A.

REFERENCE

Pick, J. R., R. A. Goyer, J. B. Graham, and J. H. Renwick. 1967. Subluxation of the carpus in dogs. An X chromosome defect closely linked with the locus for hemophilia A. Lab. Invest. 17:243–48.

CERVICAL VERTEBRAL DEFORMITY (Wobbler Syndrome)

Cervical vertebral deformation with pressure on the spinal cord and resultant weakness and ataxia has been reported in the Great Dane, basset, Doberman pinscher, Rhodesian Ridgeback, Saint Bernard, Irish setter, fox terrier, and English sheepdog. Clinical signs may progress from partial paraplegia to total quadriplegia. Signs of incoordination may be present at birth, but signs usually first occur between 3 and 12 months of age. Hind limbs are affected, followed in some dogs by the

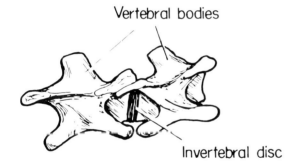

Fig. 5.2. *Canine vertebrae. The intervertebral disc, composed of a pliable center (nucleus pulposus) with a tough enveloping membrane (annulus fibrosis), is situated between successive vertebrae and serves as a shock absorber as well as to maintain flexibility in the axial skeleton.*

forelimbs. Rear limb incoordination, hypermetria (a prancing gait), or dragging of the feet may occur.

Two types of deformity can usually be demonstrated by radiographs of the affected part in flexion. In the first type there is a slight subluxation, with narrowing of the spinal canal. This type most often affects the midcervical region. The second type of cervical spondylolisthesis (dislocation) usually is more caudal and has a prominent feature of altered vertebral body shape and articulation. Narrowing of the spinal canal is usually obvious both in Danes and in Dobermans. In the Great Dane the vertebral defect occurs at approximately cervical vertebrae 5-6 or 6-7 and was described as an overriding of the cranial epiphysis of one vertebra on the caudal epiphysis of the immediately adjacent vertebra. (Upward tilting of one vertebra and a downward tilting of another causes a narrowing of the canal between the two.) The compression of the spinal cord results first in ataxia of the hind limbs, which gradually progresses to involve the forelimbs.

In some cases, at the site of compression, necrosis of the gray matter was noted as well as Wallerian degeneration in the white matter above and below the pressure site. Abnormalities in the affected vertebrae were noted.

Deformation and displacement of vertebrae may result from the effect of abnormal forces on the spine or an imbalance in conformation. The weight of the head, the length of the neck, and the muscles and the ligaments in the area are involved. In the basset a similar defect occurred at approximately cervical vertebrae 2-3, in the Ridgeback at approximately 3-4, and in the Doberman at approximately 3-4.

Inheritance and Recommendation

Pedigree studies of affected dogs (bassets) suggest some form of genetic transmission. There was a high inbreeding coefficient for affected animals. Evidence for X linkage was suggested. In one study the condition appeared to be transmitted as a recessive.

Additional information would be needed for firm recommendations. Sex-linked traits could be approached as described under sections on hemophilia A and B in Chapter 2. Recessive traits are outlined in Chapter 1.

REFERENCES

Dueland, R., R. W. Furneaux, and M. M. Kaye. Spinal fusion and dorsal lamenectomy for midcervical spondylolisthesis in a dog. JAVMA 162:366-69.
Gage, E. D., and B. F. Hoerlein. 1973. Surgical repair of cervical subluxation and spondylolisthesis in the dog. JAAHA 9:385-90.
Geary, J. C. 1969. Canine spinal lesions not involving discs. JAVMA 155:2038-46.

La Croix, J. A. 1970. Diagnosis of orthopedic problems peculiar to the growing dog. Vet. Med. Small Anim. Clin. 65:229–36.

Palmer, A. C., and M. E. Wallace. 1967. Deformation of cervical vertebrae in basset hounds. Vet. Rec. 80:430–33.

Selcer, R. R., and J. E. Olina. 1975. Cervical spondylopathy: Wobbler syndrome in dogs. JAAHA 11:175–79.

Wolvekamp, W. T., and G. H. Wentink. 1975. Vertebral body deformation causing wobbler syndrome in a Great Dane. Tijdschr. Diergeneeskd. 100(14):775–80.

Wright, F., J. R. Rest, and A. C. Palmer. 1973. Ataxia of the Great Dane caused by stenosis of the cervical vertebral canal: Comparison with similar conditions in the basset hound, Doberman pinscher, Ridgeback, and the Thoroughbred Horse. Vet. Rec. 92:1–6.

CRANIOSCHISIS (Skull Fissures)

Cranioschisis refers to a persistent soft spot in the skull and has been reported in one family of cocker spaniels. Pups usually do not live more than a few weeks.

Under normal conditions the cranial sutures of a newborn pup are reported to be extremely small and can be detected only upon close examination. In the case reported, the cranial crevice or soft spot was about 1/8 inch wide and 1/4 inch long and, instead of disappearing shortly after birth, remained open or increased in size.

Defective skulls are apparently developmental calvarium defects or pathologic (persistent) fontanelles.

Inheritance and Recommendation

This trait was reported to be inherited as a recessive and could thus be eliminated from a kennel as outlined previously.

Select against this gene as for any recessive gene.

REFERENCE

Pullig, T. 1952. Inheritance of a skull defect in cocker spaniels. J. Hered. 43:97–99.

DWARFISM—CHONDRODYSPLASIA WITH ANEMIA (Alaskan Malamute)

Chondrodysplasia is inherited as a recessive. The front limbs of the affected dog are usually shorter than the back limbs so that the topline slopes forward. The forelegs are deformed by enlargement of the carpal joints, lateral deviation of the carpus (paw), and marked bowing of the radius (forelimbs) and ulna. Variation in severity exists.

Radiographically, the defect appears to involve the entire skeletal system, except for the skull. The greatest effect appears to be on the distal ulna and radius. The epiphyseal plates of both the ulna and radius are wide and irregular. The distal metaphysis of the radius is sclerotic and slightly mushroomed. Within the metaphysis of the ulna and extending into the diaphysis there are focal areas of decreasing density, which give these areas a rather moth-eaten appearance. The condition appears to result from impaired growth of bones in which endochondral ossification occurs. There is a gross thickening of the growth plate without loss of the regular columns of cartilage cells and apparent impairment of the conversion of cartilage to bone. The condition has been classified as chondrodysplasia.

The dwarfism is associated with erythrocyte macrocytosis and mild anemia.

Inheritance and Recommendation

Clinically, the defect is expressed as an autosomal recessive. Hematologic studies show that the heterozygote can be detected, so from this standpoint the condition appears to be incompletely dominant.

Remove affected animals from the kennel. Test mate or have blood studies conducted to determine carriers.

REFERENCES

Fletch, S. M., and P. H. Pinkerton. 1972. An inherited anemia associated with hereditary chondrodysplasia in the Alaskan malamute. Can. Vet. J. 13:270–71.

_____. 1973. Animal models of human disease. Congenital hemolytic anemia: Inherited hemolytic anemia with stomatocytosis in the Alaskan malamute dog. Am. J. Pathol. 71:477–80.

Fletch, S. M., P. H. Pinkerton, and P. J. Brueckner. 1975. The Alaskan malamute chondrodysplasia (dwarfism-anemia) syndrome in review. JAAHA 11:353–61.

Smart, M. E., and S. M. Fletch. 1971. A hereditary skeletal growth defect in purebred Alaskan malamutes. (Letters to Editor.) Can. Vet. J. 12:31–32.

Subden, R. E. 1972. Genetics of the Alaskan malamute chondrodysplasia syndrome. J. Hered. 63:149–52.

DWARFISM (Shetland Sheepdog)

The occurrence of dwarfism in Shetland sheepdogs has been reported. Five sheltie dwarfs have appeared in three litters from the breeding of two sons of one stud to three of his daughters. The affected dogs are disproportionate dwarfs; the dogs' bodies appear normal but their legs are short and distorted. Dogs are approximately 9 inches tall.

Inheritance and Recommendation

With limited data, the condition is believed to be transmitted as a simple recessive.

Select against this trait as for any recessive gene.

REFERENCE
Roll, M. H. 1975. A commentary on dwarfism in Shetland sheepdogs. Sheltie Special
    14(6):19–21.

HIP DYSPLASIA

Canine hip dysplasia (CHD) (*dys,* bad, and *plasia,* form)   is a
developmental disease of the hip joints. Hip dysplasia occurs in all
breeds, but the prevalence of hip dysplasia is much higher in some breeds
than in others. The true prevalence of hip dysplasia among the various
breeds is not known. Data published by the Orthopedic Foundation for
Animals (OFA) on approximately 38,000 radiographs list the following
breeds with over 25% dysplastic animals: Saint Bernard, Newfoundland,
bull mastiff, Gordon setter, Old English sheepdog, English springer
spaniel, Akita, Chesapeake Bay retriever, golden retriever, Norwegian

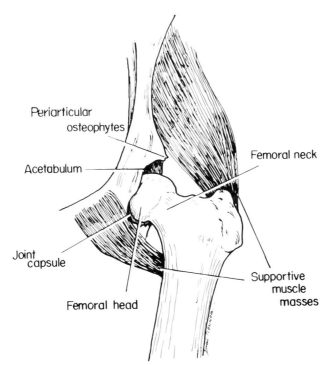

Fig. 5.3. *Canine hip joint. This is the site of hip dysplasia. The
supportive muscles and the angle of the femoral neck relate to
whether a joint is normal or dysplastic. Periarticular osteophytes
may cause pain and interfere with joint mobility.*

elkhound, Rottweiler, and German shepherd. This percentage for hip dysplasia should not be considered as absolute since it is based only on those radiographs submitted to OFA, and many radiographs were probably screened out and not submitted, and many dogs of the particular breeds are not radiographed at all. Affected pups appear to have normal hips at birth; the defect gradually develops with increasing age. The most frequent age for the appearance of hip dysplasia is approximately 5 months (with a range of 3–8 months). Two phases are involved. The first, the acute phase, occurs during the pup's rapid growing period. During this phase the dog may demonstrate pain in the hip region in various ways. It may "flop" down instead of the more normal manner of lying down more slowly; it may show difficulty in rising, etc. The second phase, a more chronic arthritic phase, occurs in the older dog. Signs of dysplasia in the dog may include restricted motion of the hip joint, self-limited exercise, lameness, and atrophy of the thigh muscles. In mature dogs symptoms may lessen or disappear, or some dogs will show minimal, if any, discomfort or malfunction.

Pathophysiology

Hip dysplasia is a deformity of the coxofemoral joint or joints. It may be characterized radiographically by a shallow acetabulum (socket), flattening of the femoral head (ball), coxofemoral subluxation (separation), or secondary degenerative joint disease. This condition represents or results from a disparity between primary muscle mass and too rapid growth of the skeleton. The muscle fails to develop or at least lags behind skeletal development. This lack of muscle or muscle mass that the joint should depend on for stability allows separation or pulling apart. This separation triggers the events that are called hip dysplasia or degenerative joint disease. As a result, the femoral head fails to seat properly in the socket. When contact is not full and constant, abnormalities occur in the shape of the socket and later to the femoral head. The acetabulum shifts from a deep socket to a shallow groove (fills with bone). The femoral head flattens and fails to seat. Abnormal wear with erosion of the joint cartilage occurs, and the result is the thickening of the joint capsule and formation of periarticular osteophytes (spurs).

The only defects found on close observation are soft tissue defects. These include a lack of muscle mass and connective tissue. Bony changes of the hip occur because the soft tissues do not have sufficient strength to maintain congruity between the articular surface of the femoral head and the acetabulum. The changes in bone merely reflect changes in the cartilage and supporting tissue. Hip dysplasia develops only if hip joint stability and joint incongruity occur together. Therefore, the changes in cartilage and bone may be considered by some as secondary. Cartilage abnormalities are regularly observed in affected dogs and not with most normal individuals.

Inheritance

Hip joint conformation is not an all or none phenomenon. That is, it is not either "normal" or "dysplastic." Hip joint conformation is a continuum from good to bad and all shades in between. Hip joint status is usually classified as excellent, good, fair, mild CHD, moderate CHD, or severe CHD.

This variation in dogs and among littermates is suggestive of a polygenetic pattern or multigenic nature. In the German shepherd a heritability index of approximately 0.25 was reported. This means that the defect is under genetic control, but the environment under which the dog is maintained influences the expression of the trait. Predisposing factors include growth rate, body type, and pelvic muscle mass.

Recommendation

One should strongly consider breeding only dogs having radiographically normal hips, unless other qualities of an individual dog dictate differently. Other traits must always be considered. The prevalence of dysplasia dogs in studies has been reduced by selective breeding.

REFERENCES

Cardinett, G. H., M. M. Guffy, and L. J. Wallace. 1974. Canine hip dysplasia. Effects of pectineal tenotomy on the coxofemoral joints of German shepherd dogs. JAVMA 164:591–98.

Larsen, J. S., and E. A. Corley. 1971. Radiographic evaluations in a canine hip dysplasia control program. JAVMA 159:989–92.

Lust, G. 1974. Pathogenesis of degenerative hip joint disease in young dogs. Gaines Dog Research (Progress), Winter 1974, pp. 4–5.

Orthopedic Foundation for Animals, Inc. 1973. Canine hip dysplasia. Proceedings of the Canine Hip Dysplasia Symposium and Workshop, St. Louis, Mo.

Pharr, J. W., and J. P. Morgan. 1976. Hip dysplasia in Australian shepherd dogs. JAAHA 12(4):439–45.

Riser, W. H. 1974. Canine hip dysplasia: Cause and control. JAVMA 164:360–62.

Riser, W. H., and J. S. Larsen. 1974. Influence of breed somatotypes on prevalence of hip dysplasia in the dog. JAVMA 166:79–81.

Riser, W. H., and H. Miller. 1966. Canine hip dysplasia and how to control it. Orthopedic Foundation for Animals, Inc., and Hip Dysplasia Control Registry, P. O. Box 8251, Philadelphia, Pa. 19101.

Schnelle, G. B. 1973. The present status and outlook on canine hip dysplasia. Gaines Dog Research (Progress), Spring 1973, pp. 1–6.

PATELLAR LUXATION

Patellar luxation is an abnormality frequently observed in the smaller breeds of dogs. Other deformities may also occur with the luxation syndrome. Although luxation of the patella may occur in larger breeds as the result of trauma, the high incidence of congenital luxation in breeds such as the miniature poodle, Chihuahua, Boston terrier, toy fox terrier, Pekingese, cocker spaniel, schnauzer, King Charles, Cavalier spaniel, Yorkshire terrier, Shetland "collie," Pomeranian, griffon, Japanese spaniel, and French bulldog suggests an inherited characteristic and a man-made defect. Luxations usually are first reported in the young, growing dog at 4–6 months of age.

Luxations are usually medial and may be unilateral or bilateral. Luxations may be recurrent or complete. Severity of the defect varies considerably from minor soft tissue damage to marked bony malformation with severe secondary soft tissue abnormalities; from recurrent subluxation of the patella, with little functional problems, to a state where the joint is fixed and the animal moves in a crouched position.

The normal function of the patella and possible causes for luxation have been described in the literature as follows: the patella is a small bone that articulates with the trochlea at the distal end of the femur and plays a subsidiary role in the extensor mechanism of the stifle joint. It functions mainly in protecting the patellar ligament from frictional damage during the acts of extension and flexion of the joint. The quadriceps muscle and the patellar ligament are inserted from the other components of the extensor apparatus.

In a voluntary act of extension of the stifle joint from a flexed position, the quadriceps femoris muscle is contracted. This force of contraction of the muscle is relayed through the patella and its ligament to the anterior tibial tuberosity. The upward pull on the anterior tibial tuberosity brings about the extension of the femorotibial articulation. In a normal joint the direction of the force of contraction of the quadriceps muscle, the femoral trochlea, and the anterior tibial tuberosity is practically in alignment and this helps to confine the patella to the femoral trochlea in its upward movements during acts of extension of the joint. The balanced tension of capsular attachments in the medial and lateral aspects of the patella and the prominent nature of the ridges on the lateral and medial sides of the femoral trochlea further prevent the patella from being dislodged in either medial or lateral direction during these acts of extension of the joint. As opposed to this, the slimy consistency of the joint synovia and resultant force acting on the patella in the direction of the trochlea would facilitate a luxation of the patella if the conditions that help to maintain the patella in the trochlea are altered in any way.

Any of the following could cause luxation:

1. If the direction of the force of contraction of the quadriceps muscle is out of alignment with the rest of extensor apparatus.

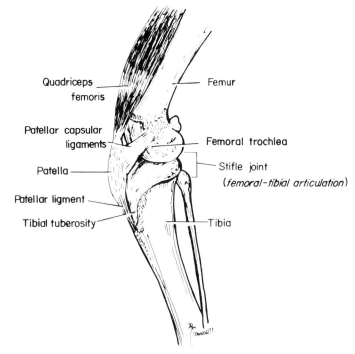

Fig. 5.4. *Canine stifle joint. Note the relationships of patellar ligaments and quadriceps muscle to the patella. The patella functions through and is held in place by proper attachment.*

2. If the femoral trochlea is out of alignment.

3. If the anterior tibial tuberosity is displaced to a more medial or lateral position on the tibia.

4. If the degree of concavity of the femoral trochlear groove and the degree of prominence of the femoral trochlear ridge are reduced in any way.

5. If the balance of tension between the medial and lateral aspects of the capsular attachment of the patella is upset in any way.

Displacement of the patella from its normal position alters the direction of force of the quadriceps muscle contraction acting on the patellar displacement.

Inheritance and Recommendation

The literature suggests that this condition is the result of a recessive or polygenic type of gene action. The condition occurs in both sexes.

A selective breeding program should be followed. All affected animals should be eliminated. Then select as outlined against recessive genes.

REFERENCES

DeAngelis, M. 1971. Patellar luxation in dogs. Vet. Clin. North Am. 1:403–5.

Hodgman, S. F. J. 1963. Abnormalities and defects in pedigree dogs. 1. An investigation into the existence of abnormalities in pedigree dogs in the British Isles. J. Small Anim. Pract. 4:447–56.

Horne, R. D. 1971. Canine patellar luxation. (A review.) Vet. Med. Small Anim. Clin. 66:211–18.

Hutt, F. B. 1968. Genetic defects of bones and joints in domestic animals. Cornell Vet. 58 (Suppl.):104–13.

Kaplan, B. 1971. Surgical palliation of bilateral congenital medial patellar luxation. Vet. Med. Small Anim. Clin. 66:571–74.

Knight, G. C. 1963. Abnormalities and defects in pedigree dogs. 3. Tibio-femoral joint deformity and patellar luxation. J. Small Anim. Pract. 4:463–64.

Kodituwakku, G. E. 1962. Luxation of the patella in the dog. Vet. Rec. 74:1499–1507.

Nesuke, E. I., et al. 1968. Patellar looseness: Significance, treatment, and prognosis. Mod. Vet. Pract. 47(4):54–59.

Priester, W. A. 1972. Sex, age, and breed as risk factors in canine patellar dislocation. JAVMA 160:740–42.

Priester, W. A., A. G. Glass, and N. S. Waggoner. 1970. Congenital defects in domesticated animals: General considerations. Am. J. Vet. Res. 31:1871–79.

Rudy, R. L. 1966. Inheritance of patellar anomalies in dogs. Mod. Vet. Pract. 47(1):54.

Shuttleworth, A. C. 1935. Dislocation of the patella in the dog. Vet. Rec. 15:765–74.

Singleton, W. B. 1957. The diagnosis and treatment of some abnormal stifle conditions in the dog. Vet. Rec. 69:1387–98.

———. 1961. Differential diagnosis of stifle injuries in the dog. J. Small Anim. Pract. 1:182–91.

POLYDACTYLY (Dew Claw)

The presence of dew claws (one or more extra digits on toes) is common in many breeds and, unless removed, could cause some difficulty.

Apparently the dew claw or extra toe represents a reappearance of the first digit lost during evolution in most Canidae.

Dew claws are usually removed soon after birth with very little difficulty, so selection against the dew claw is not usually considered of prime importance.

Inheritance

Dew claws (back leg) are generally believed to be inherited as a dominant, however, at least one report on one breed states that dew claws are recessively inherited.

REFERENCES

Falaschini, A. 1941. On the mode of inheritance of dew claws in the domestic dog. Nuova. Vet. 19:126.

Grundmann, I. 1954. The inheritance of polydactyly in the domestic dog. Vet. Med. Diss. Frei. Univ. Berlin.

Keeler, C. E., and H. C. Trimble. 1938. The inheritance of dew claws in the dog. J. Hered. 19:145–48.

Kelly, R. B. 1949. Sheep Dogs: Their Breeding, Maintenance, and Training. Sydney: Angus and Robertson.

Whitney, L. F. 1948. How to Breed Dogs. New York: Orange Judd.

POLYOSTOTIC FIBROUS DYSPLASIA

Bone cysts are rare in the dog. The condition may be inherited or at least it has been reported in closely related Doberman pinschers. The cystic bone condition occurs in the distal metaphyses of the radius and/or ulna. The condition first becomes apparent at 4–7 months of age. Enlarged swollen areas in the region of the cyst and occasional pain and lameness may be observed. Fracture is common at the site of the bone cyst.

The bone cyst is an osteolytic defect usually near the epiphysis. Bone is replaced by fibrous tissue that may contain areas of cystic degeneration. The honeycombed single cavity of the cyst is lined with a smooth, thin, fibrous connective tissue membrane and is usually filled with straw-colored fluid that on occasion might contain blood.

Cystic areas show well-defined borders with a marked thinning of the overlying cortices. The diameter of the shaft appears to be increased locally. The thinning of the cortex can be seen to have taken place from the medullary interior surface. The periosteal surface is smooth, with absence of activity or new bone formation except in the region of fracture repair. The cortical walls consist of loose osseous tissue containing a number of osteoclasts or bone-absorbing cells.

Inheritance and Recommendation

It has been suggested that the condition was inherited and possibly was due to a recessive gene.

The condition is rare, but if it should occur in any breed, avoid the mating of close relatives in a breeding program.

REFERENCES

B.S.A.V.A. Orthopaedic Group. 1967. J. Small Anim. Pract. 8:649–53.

Carrig, C. B., and Seawright, A. A. 1967. A familial canine polyostotic fibrous dysplasia with subperiosteal cortical defects. J. Small Anim. Pract. 10:391–405.

Gourley, J., and D. W. Eden. 1954. Bone cyst in a dog. Vet. Rec. 66:63.

Huff, R. W., and R. S. Brodey. 1964. Multiple bone cysts in a dog: A case report. J. Am. Vet. Radiol. Soc. 5:40–46.

Owen, L. N. 1967. Calcinosis circumscripta (calcium gout) in related Irish wolfhounds. J. Small Anim. Pract. 8:291–92.

Seawright, A. A., and L. R. Grono. 1961. Calcinosis circumscripta in dogs. Aust. Vet. J. 37:421–25.

OVERSHOT (Prognathia) AND UNDERSHOT (Retrognathia) JAW

Structural abnormalities of the canine skull are frequently observed. Two of the more noticeable defects are overshot (prognathia) and undershot (retrognathia) jaw.

Although the terms prognathia and retrognathia can refer to either the maxillae or mandible or both, they are usually used in describing the mandible or lower jaw. Both of these defects are believed to be genetically influenced. The undershot condition is more common in the short-headed breeds such as the bulldog, Pekingese, and Boston terrier. The overshot jaw (pig jaw) is more common in the long-headed breeds. In certain breeds these abnormalities are selected for as a desirable breed characteristic.

A condition in which the mandible is too short in proportion to the upper jaw (overshot) has been reported in long-haired dachshunds and cocker spaniels. Cocker pups may appear normal at birth, and even at weaning, but show the defect at maturity. Great variations in the expression of this trait exist.

With the long-haired dachshund, the animal appears to have a somewhat longer and more pointed nose than the normal dog. From a side view, the upper lip droops and hangs down over the mandible. This drooping of the upper lip may be recognized in the newborn pup. When one retracts the lips from the teeth, an abnormal occlusion of the teeth may be observed. There is no contact between the upper and lower incisors. Alteration develops in the position of the teeth. Apparently the defect involves only the anterior part of the mandible. The alteration observed in the upper jaw teeth is secondary in nature due to the alteration in pressure.

Inheritance and Recommendation

The trait appears inherited as a recessive with multiple modifying factors in the cocker. Long-haired dachshunds show a similar autosomal recessive character. In a genetic study concerning the variations of the canine skull, length of jaw and the relation of jaw length to other skull characteristics and deformities were examined in crosses of long-headed and short-headed breeds. It was concluded that long maxillas and long mandibles were due to multiple factors and that those factors conditioning a long jaw were imperfectly dominant over a short jaw with the dominance better expressed in the lower than the upper jaw. The genes determining length of upper and lower jaws appear to be inherited independently of each other.

Select against this trait as outlined for any recessive. Always consider traits may be inherited differently in different breeds.

REFERENCES

Gruneberg, H., and A. J. Lea. 1940. An inherited jaw anomaly in long-haired dachshunds. J. Genet. 39:285–96.

Phillips, J. McI. 1945. Pig jaw in the cocker spaniels: Retrognathia of the mandible in the cocker spaniel and its relationship to other deformities of the jaw. J. Hered. 36:177-81.

Stockard, C. R. 1941. The genetic and endocrine basis for differences in form and behavior as elucidated by studies of contrasted pure-line dog breeds and their hybrids. Am. Anat. Memoirs, 19. Philadelphia: Wistar Institute of Anatomy and Biology.

SHORT SPINE (Spina Bifida)

A short-spined condition has been observed in native Japanese dogs, mixed dogs of the Japanese cross, and in beagles selectively bred for short tails. Similar cases have been reported in dogs in various parts of the world.

Great variations in phenotype occur, but in studies involving more than one individual dog the following summarizes most cases. The entire spinal column is short when compared to the lengths of the head and legs, giving the dog an apelike appearance. The shoulders are high and the back slopes sharply toward the tail. The trunk is somewhat crooked and the dog has a screw-shaped or kinky tail.

Pathophysiology

Axial skeletal defects are produced through abnormal induction of the sclerotome by segmental defects of the notochord. In the greyhound, the anomaly is due to a progressive expression of sclerotome inhibition, resulting in vertebral malformation and impaction.

Inheritance and Recommendation

The condition in Japanese dogs is presumably hereditary, but the type of gene action is not given. The condition in greyhounds was reported to be autosomal recessive. Apparently the condition in beagles is due to an autosomal dominant gene with reduced penetrance and variable expressivity.

Since the condition is rare, no problem should exist. If the trait as suggested in beagles is dominant, remove affected animals.

REFERENCES

Curtis, R. L., D. English, and Y. J. Kim. 1964. Spina bifida in "stub" dog stocks selectively bred for short tails. Anat. Rec. 148:365.

De Boom, H. P. A. 1965. Anomalous animals. South African J. Sci. 61:159-71.

Hansen, H. J. 1968. Historical evidence of an unusual deformity in dogs (short-spine dog). J. Small Anim. Pract. 9:163-68.

Kalter, H. 1968. Teratology of the central nervous system. Chicago and London: University of Chicago Press.

Suu, S. 1956. Studies in the short-spine dog. I. Their origin and occurrence. Res. Bull. Fac. Agric. Gifu Univ. 7:127-34.

Suu, S., and T. Ueshima. 1957. Studies in the short-spine dog. II. Somatological observations. Res. Bull. Fac. Agric. Gifu Univ. 8:112-28.

UNUNITED ANCONEAL PROCESS (Elbow Dysplasia)

Ununited anconeal process is an orthopedic disease of young dogs resulting in the failure of normal fusion of the anconeal process to the diaphysis of the ulna. The condition may occur bilaterally or unilaterally. This condition is also referred to as elbow dysplasia, but the term *elbow dysplasia* includes other anomalies. Clinical signs vary between individual dogs and may not become noticeable until the dog approaches 8 months of age. One observation is continuous or intermittently mild to severe lameness due to the loose piece of bone in the elbow joint and possible secondary osteoarthritis. Other signs include distention of the joint capsule, crepitation (sound of bone rubbing), decreased extension and flexion, and lateral deviation of the elbow (winging out) during movement or while standing (may toe outward with spread digits). Secondary complications such as osteoarthritis and disuse atrophy involving muscles may occur.

This condition is believed to be hereditary and is found more frequently in the German shepherd, basset hound, French bulldog, Saint Bernard, Great Dane, Labrador retriever, bull mastiff, Irish wolfhound,

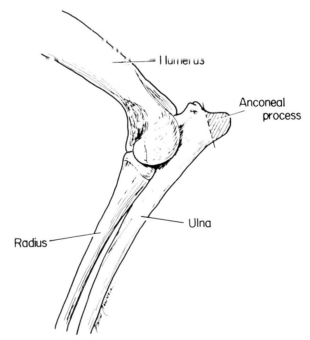

Fig. 5.5. *Canine elbow joint. The anconeal process and the radius serve as attachment points for the muscles of extension and flexion. Malalignment of this joint may result in an abnormal gait and eventual excessive wear in the joint.*

pointer, blood hound, Great Pyrenees, Weimaraner, dachshund, and Newfoundland.

Digital palpation of the elbow may result in pain in some cases. Early cases may show synovial swelling just caudal to the lateral condyle of the humerus. There may be some thickening of the joint capsule both laterally and medially on the elbow joint and crepitus may be indicated during flexion and severe extension of the elbow. As the problem becomes chronic, the increased synovial swelling may disappear, more crepitus may be detected, and muscular atrophy of the triceps and biceps due to disease may be noted.

Final diagnosis is confirmed by radiograph. The anconeal process in large breeds of dogs has been shown by some to develop from a separate center of ossification. This center appears at 93 ± 11 days and unites with the ulnar diaphysis at 124 ± 17 days. A diagnosis of ununited anconeal process prior to this age is unwarranted. Nonunion or a partial union results in a loose portion of bone within the elbow joint that acts as a foreign body and irritant causing lameness and arthritis.

Inheritance and Recommendation

Based on a limited number of nonrandomly selected dogs, a dominant multiple (3-gene pair) type of inheritance has been suggested, with some reservations, for elbow dysplasia.

Affected dogs should not be used for breeding purposes.

REFERENCES

Bradney, I. W. 1967. Non-union of the anconeal process in the dog. Aust. Vet. J. 43:215–16.

Campbell, J. R. 1971. Luxation and ligamentous injuries of the elbow of the dog. Vet. Clin. North Am. 1:429–40.

Carlson, W. D., and G. Severin. 1961. Elbow dysplasia in the dog: A preliminary report. JAVMA 138:295–97.

Cawley, A. J., and J. Archibald. 1959. Ununited anconeal processes of the dog. JAVMA 134:454–58.

Clarkson, A. R., and B. H. Lunn. 1970. Ununited anconeal process (elbow dysplasia) in a dog. New Zealand Vet. J. 18:91–94.

Corley, E. A., and W. D. Carlson. 1965. Radiographic, genetic, and pathologic aspects of elbow dysplasia. JAVMA 147:1651.

Corley, E. A., W. D. Carlson, T. M. Sutherland, J. A. Flint, and H. N. Newkirk. 1963. Elbow dysplasia: A genetic and pathologic study. Annual Report, AM06597–01, U.S. Department of Health, Education and Welfare, Public Health Service, Washington, D.C.

Corley, E. A., T. M. Sutherland, and W. D. Carlson. 1968. Genetic aspects of canine elbow dysplasia. JAVMA 153:543–47.

Fox, M. W. 1964. Polyarthodysplasia (congenital joint luxation) in the dog. JAVMA 145:1204–5.

Hanlon, G. F. 1969. Additional radiographic observations on elbow dysplasia in the dog. JAVMA 155:2045–46.

Hare, W. C. D. 1962. Congenital detachment of the processus anconeus in the dog. Vet. Rec. 74:545–46.

Herron, M. R. 1969. Ununited anconeal process: Diagnosis and therapy. Southwest. Vet., Summer 1969, pp. 267–71.

_____. 1971. Ununited anconeal process in the dog. Vet. Clin. North Am. 1(3):417–28.

Ljunggren, G., A. J. Cawley, and J. Archibald. 1966. Elbow dysplasia in the dog. JAVMA 148:887–90.

Stiern, R. A. 1956. Ectopic sesamoid bones at the elbow (patella cubiti) of the dog. JAVMA 128:498–501.

Stevens, D. R., and R. D. Sande. 1974. An elbow dysplasia syndrome in the dog. JAVMA 165:1065–69.

Ticer, J. W. 1973. Radiographic interpretation. Mod. Vet. Pract. 54:37–42.

Van Sickle, D. C. 1966. Relationship of ossification to canine elbow dysplasia. Anim. Hosp. 2:24–31.

Vaughan, L. D. 1962. Congenital detachment of the processus anconeus in the dog. Vet. Rec. 74:309–11.

CHAPTER 6

Neuromuscular System

ATAXIA

A hereditary cerebellar ataxia has been observed in smooth-haired fox terriers in Sweden. A similar clinical disease has been reported in one French bulldog, a Scottish terrier, two Boston terriers, and the Airedale. In the fox terrier the disease becomes noticeable at approximately 2½–4 months of age. Clinical signs include restlessness, unusual barking and howling, and rubbing the head against objects.

The condition is progressive, with intervals of stationary symptoms and with eventual varying difficulty of movement. Dogs may fall with slight changes of position and experience difficulty in rising. The condition does not cause death.

Pathophysiology

In five fox terriers examined histologically, there was bilateral demyelination in the cervical, thoracic, and lumbar parts of the spinal cord in the region of the posterior and peripheral parts of the lateral white columns and the medial parts of the anterior white columns. Demyelination changes were in two groups of fibers. One group lies bilaterally in the extreme peripheral region of the posteriolateral part of the lateral white columns extending anteriorally from the posterior horns (posterior spinocerebellar tract). The other group lies in the most medial part of the anterior white column just adjacent to the anterior median fissure.

Inheritance and Recommendation

The ataxia described for the fox terrier was genetically dependent. It was found to result from a recessive, autosomal gene.

Dogs showing the condition should not be used for breeding. Test mating from carrier animals could be made to detect other carriers.

REFERENCES

Bjorck, G., S. Dyrendahl, and S. E. Olsson. 1957. Hereditary ataxia in smooth-haired fox terriers. Vet. Rec. 69:871–76.

Bjorck, G., W. Mar, S. G. Olsson, and P. Sourander. 1962. Hereditary ataxia in fox terriers. Acta Neuropathol. Suppl. I, 45–48.

Saunders, L. Z. 1952. A checklist of hereditary and familial diseases of the central nervous system in domestic animals. Cornell Vet. 42:592–600.

EPILEPSY

Epilepsy may result from injury to the head, metabolic disease, or many other causes but is often due to unknown (idiopathic) causes. Evidence of an inherited epilepsy in the dog is convincing. The term epilepsy means recurring episodic seizures (convulsions, fits). This condition of generalized convulsions is observed in most domestic animals, but apparently there is a greater frequency in the dog than in the other species. In some reports this disorder accounted for approximately 1% of all canine diseases diagnosed. Epilepsy has been observed in many breeds including the Scottish terrier, springer spaniel, poodle, Pomeranian, Pekingese, Chihuahua, German shepherd, Chesapeake Bay retriever, Boston terrier, collie, Belgian Tervuren, Keeshond, beagle, Welsh corgi, pointer, setter, boxer, dachshund, Saint Bernard, Great Dane, Airedale, retriever, Siberian husky, Shetland sheepdog, bloodhound, and Lhaso Apso. A strong suggestion for an inherited epilepsy or at least an inherited predisposition to seizures has been found for the dachshund, beagle, collie, Keeshond, German shepherd, cocker spaniel, miniature poodle, and Tervuren as well as setters, retrievers, and spaniels. The first seizure usually occurs between the ages of 6 months and 3 years.

It is now believed that in the dog partial epilepsies (psychomotor) have a high incidence and perhaps a genetic background. Clinical signs include anxiety, fear, masticatory movement, and automatism (nonreflex acts without conscious volition). This type of epilepsy may in time develop into the generalized form. Clinical signs for this generalized type of epilepsy include aura; i.e., prior to actual seizure the dog may approach his owner and whine or whimper. The animal loses consciousness suddenly and falls. Muscle spasm (tonus) affects the entire body. Intermittent relaxation occurs with a paddling movement of the legs. Involuntary urination, defecation, and frothing at the mouth may be observed.

This condition usually will be experienced for less than 5 minutes. For a period of hours thereafter the dog may appear disoriented. The frequency of convulsions varies from several per day to one or two a year. All signs may not be observed in an individual animal.

Pathophysiology

Epilepsy is a disorder or malfunction of the brain. The seizures observed are the clinical expressions for a state produced by an abnormal excessive neuronal discharge within the central nervous system. Etiologic factors include abnormal neurons acting as pacemakers. Defective inhibitory controls in symmetric circuitry alter the neurochemical environment of neurons. In one report, inclusion bodies did occur in glial and neuronal cells in the brain in dogs with a familial form of epilepsy (beagles). In this report histologic changes were also observed in other organs.

Inheritance

The exact mode of the inheritance of this predisposition is not well documented. It has been suggested that at least for the German shepherd, collie, and Keeshond epilepsy results from a single autosomal recessive gene. In one study with beagles a difference was observed between sexes, with a higher incidence in males. Two possible genetic hypotheses (a single sex-linked recessive and a simple autosomal recessive) were considered, and neither completely fit the reported data. A genetic hypothesis utilizing two loci (one an autosomal recessive and the other a sex-linked suppressor) was advanced. Further evidence is needed. In a study made with the British Alsatian (German shepherd) the following was concluded: The trait has a genetic base; it is sex modified—as with the beagle, a higher incidence (3.6–1) was observed for males. More than one gene is believed to be involved and these genes interrelate in an additive manner. A higher incidence in male Keeshonden has been reported. It was also observed in some studies that electroencephalographic coding has little or no relation to fits.

Recommendation

Since the expression of this trait may be somewhat latent, breeding tests would not be practical. Select against this gene by not using animals or their close relatives that exhibit the trait.

REFERENCES

Barker, J. 1973. Epilepsy in the dog: A comparative approach. J. Small Anim. Pract. 14:281–89.

Bielfelt, S. W., H. C. Redman, and R. D. McClellon. 1971. Sire-sex related differences in rates of epileptiform seizures in a purebred beagle dog colony. Am. J. Vet. Res. 32:2039–49.

Croft, P. G. 1962. The EEG as an aid to diagnosis of nervous disease in the dog and cat. J. Small Anim. Pract. 3:205–13.

_____. 1965. Fits in dogs: A survey of 260 cases. Vet. Rec. 77:439–45.

_____. 1968. The use of the electroencephalograph in the detection of epilepsy as a hereditary condition in the dog. Vet. Rec. 88:712–13.

_____. 1971. Fits in dogs. Vet. Rec. 88:118–20.

Croft, P. G., and M. J. R. Stockman. 1963. Epilepsy in the Keeshond. Vet. Rec. 75:36.

_____. 1964. Inherited defects in dogs. Vet. Rec. 76:260–61.

Cunningham, J. G. 1971. Canine seizure disorders. JAVMA 158:589–97.

Eberhart, G. W. 1951. Epilepsy in the dog. Gaines Symp., pp. 18–20.

Falco, M. J., J. Barker, and M. E. Wallace. 1974. The genetics of epilepsy in the British Alsatian. J. Small Anim. Pract. 15:685–92.

Fox, M. W. 1966. Canine disease of possible hereditary origin. Mod. Vet. Pract. 42:51–54.

Hegreberg, G. A., and G. A. Padgett. 1976. Inherited progressive epilepsy of the dog with comparisons to Lafora's disease of man. Fed. Proc. 35:1202–5.

Holliday, T. A., J. G. Cunningham, and J. J. Gutnick. 1970. Comparative clinical and electroencephalographic studies of canine epilepsy. Epilepsia 11:281–92.

Lawler, D. C. 1971. Epilepsy in dogs. New Zealand Vet. J. 19:53.

Oliver, J. E., Jr., and B. F. Hoelein. 1965. Convulsive disorders of dogs. JAVMA 146(10):1126–33.

Palmer, A. C. 1972. Pathological changes in the brain associated with fits in dogs. Vet. Rec. 90:167–72.

Parker, A. J. 1963. Epilepsy in the dog: Causes, classification, and diagnosis. Illinois Vet. 16:5–10.

Redman, H. C., and J. E. Weir. 1969. Detection of naturally occurring neurologic disorders of beagle dogs by electroencephalography. Am. J. Vet. Res. 30:2075.

Van Der Velden, N. A. 1968. Fits in Tervuren shepherd dogs. A presumed hereditary trait. J. Small Anim. Pract. 63:70.

Wallace, M. E. 1975. Keeshonds: A genetic study of epilepsy and EEG readings. J. Small Anim. Pract. 16:1–10.

FAMILIAL AMAUROTIC IDIOCY (G$_{M2}$ Gangliosidosis)

A ganglioside storage disease has been observed in the German shorthaired pointer. At approximately 6 months of age pups exhibit increased nervousness and a decreased ability or responsiveness to training. By 9–12 months, locomotor disability or ataxia is apparent and seizures are occasionally observed. Neurologic impairment progresses to decreased vision and occasional blindness, deafness, and stupor, with death occurring by 2 years of age.

Pathophysiology

Histopathologic lesions affect almost all central neurons that contain granular material in their cytoplasm. The accumulation (neuronal deposition) of G$_{M2}$ (principal storage lipid in dogs) results in an enlargement. In diseased dogs, ganglioside NANA in cerebral gray matter was increased 3.5–4.0 times normal and G$_{M2}$ ganglioside accounted for 60%–65% of the ganglioside. The gangliosides in the liver increased 3 times in affected dogs and was mainly G$_{M2}$. The accumulation probably results from an enzyme deficiency. In the dog, the enzyme defect is unknown. Based on human data, the disease would be caused by a hexosaminidase deficiency. The B-D-N-acetylgalactosaminidase activity (*p*-nitrophenyl-B-D-N acetylgalactopyranoside substrate) in tissue from diseased dogs is 3–5 times greater than normal.

Inheritance and Recommendation

Most recent evidence suggests an autosomal recessive trait. Select against as for any recessive condition.

NEURONAL CEROID-LIPOFUSCINOSIS
(Juvenile Amaurotic Familial Idiocy [AFI])

An amaurotic idiocy in the English setter was characterized by a neuronal storage of granula containing mainly insoluble PAS-positive material. A few neurons were slightly enlarged. The ganglioside content of the cerebral cortex was 1.5 times higher than found in normal animals; this could only be partly ascribed to an accumulation of ganglioside G_{M2} that might be nonspecific. In the spinal cord, the ganglioside content was twice as high as in controls, but no accumulation of any one particular ganglioside was observed.

The amaurotic idiocy of German shorthaired pointers (above section) resembles the late infantile type of G_{M2} gangliosidosis, whereas the amaurotic idiocy of English setters resembles the myoclonic variant.

Clinical signs appeared slowly. From birth to 12 months of age, most dogs with AFI show no clinical signs. First signs are dullness, decreased vision, and incoordination. As dogs grow older, signs of dullness increase. Behavior changes are more pronounced as dogs reach 15–18 months of age; they appear to lose their bearings in normal surroundings and are unable to localize sound. Signs of ataxia appear. The animals may have difficulty in locating their feed. At about 18 months of age muscular spasm may be observed. Early in the disease, an increased excitability occurs in the masseter muscle, and dogs seem cramped in the jaws and click their teeth. Later they develop tonic clonic spasms.

Histologically, both diseases are similar. Macrophages in the cerebral perivascular sheaths were not described in the English setter as in the pointer. Dogs with AFI are dehydrated and thin. The lymph glands are enlarged (2–3X). The brain (2 years old) is atrophied. Granules are found deposited in the nerve cells of 5-month-old pups. In later stages a deposition of lipid granules occurs in the nerve cells of the central nervous system, as well as in the heart, lungs, liver, and gastrointestinal tract. The cerebellum is degenerated and has glial infiltration. The Purkinje cells contain coarse lipid granules in the ganglion cells and only a small deposition in a few cells in the other layer of the retina. In peripheral nerves, demyelination and axonal degeneration are observed. The enzyme defect, if any, is not apparent. Intraneuronal lipid accumulates in the form of insoluble fluorescent lipid complexes. These lipid bodies share many characteristics with ceroid and with lipofuscin granules.

REFERENCES

Baker, H. J., J. A. Mole, J. R. Lindsey, and R. M. Creel. 1976. Animal models of human ganglioside storage disease. Fed. Proc. 35:1193–1201.

Bernheimer, H., and E. Karbe. 1970. Morphologische und neurochemische untersuchungen von 2 formen der amaurotischen idiotic der hundes. Machwers lines Gun-Gangliosidose. Acta Neuropathol. 16:243–61.

Gambetti, L. A., A. M. Kelly, and S. A. Steinberg. 1970. Biochemical studies in a canine gangliosidosis. J. Neuropathol. Exp. Neurol. 29:137–38.

Karbe, E. 1973. G_{M2} gangliosidosis (canine G_{M2} gangliosidosis) Am. J. Pathol. 71:1:151–54.

Karbe, E., and B. Schiefer. 1967. Familial amaurotic idiocy in male German shorthaired pointers. Pathol. Vet. 4:223–33.

Koppang, N. 1970. Neuronal ceroid-lipofuscinosis in English setters: Juvenile amaurotic familial idiocy (AFI) in English setters. J. Small Anim. Pract. 10:639–44.

McGrath, J. T., A. M. Kelly, and S. A. Steinberg. 1968. Cerebral lipidosis in the dog. J. Neuropathol. Exp. Neurol. 27:141.

Rac, R., and P. R. Giesecke. 1975. Lysosomal storage disease in Chihuahuas. Aust. Vet. J. 51:403–4.

GLOBOID LEUKODYSTROPHY (Krabbe Type)

Globoid leukodystrophy is a defect of galactocerebroside catabolism associated with myelin degeneration (demyelinating disorder). One observes destruction of the myelin sheath, with subsequent glial proliferation and a relative preservation of axons. The condition occurs predominantly in West Highland white and cairn terriers but has been reported in a miniature poodle, the beagle, and Bluetick hound. It is probably transmitted as an autosomal recessive. Two major syndromes are observed; one results in severe pelvic limb paralysis, in the other cerebellar signs are most common.

Clinical signs are first observed from as early as 4 weeks up to 3 months. The condition is progressive and rapid. Coordination and locomotion are primarily affected. One may initially observe weakness or loss of control of the hindquarters as well as tail tremor. Motor defects may progress to paralysis and atrophy of the muscles of the pelvic limbs. Pups may stumble, show proprioceptive defects, i.e., lack position sense of rear limbs. There is a delayed sluggish hopping reflex, limbs slide laterally, and the dog may have difficulty in standing. Cerebellar deficits are also noticed, i.e., tremors, wide stance, and incoordination. Visual deficiency may be observed and the pup may experience a loss of recognition of familiar individuals and surroundings. It may be dull and passive. Head tremors or irregular side to side and up and down head movements may be observed. Anorexia and urinary incontinence have been observed.

Pathophysiology

Lesions are restricted to the central nervous system white matter and to peripheral nerves. Histopathologically, there is diffuse degeneration of myelin sheaths accompanied by collections of globoid macrophages. Globoid cells appear vacuolated and finely granular with lacy strands of material. These globoid macrophages contain material reported to be a glycolysed (cerebroside) protein complex derived from the breakdown of myelin and may lack the ability to further process it; i.e., leukodystrophy suggests a deficiency in glial capacity to nurture or maintain myelin or degrade myelin breakdown products to fatty acids.

Initially, the globoid cells appear grouped in the perivascular space. As time progresses, the entire region of white matter is replaced by globoid cells. In the terminal stages, most of the white matter of the cerebral hemispheres is destroyed. The extent of the destruction of the white matter is varied. Within the spinal cord there appears to be preferential involvement of the dorsal and ventral roots. Patchy areas of demyelination can be found in most peripheral nerves.

In one study, dogs with globoid leukodystrophy were found to have a substantial deficiency of β-galactocerebrosidase. This enzyme normally splits galactose from galactocerebroside yielding ceramide. This results in an elevated brain cerebroside-sulfatide ratio. The deficiency of this enzyme in affected dogs is widespread—occurring in the liver and kidney as well as in the central nervous system. Therefore, this condition may be a genetically determined enzymatic disorder of myelinogenesis.

Inheritance and Recommendation

The familial pattern of this condition suggests a genetic relationship, probably a recessive.

Select as for any recessive gene where one cannot use the homozygous recessive animal in breeding.

REFERENCES

Austin, J., D. Armstrong, and G. Margolis. 1968. Canine globoid leukodystrophy: A model demyelinating disorder. Trans. Am. Neurol. Assoc. 93:181–82.

Boysen, B. G., L. Tryphonas, and N. W. Harres. 1974. Globoid cell leukodystrophy in the Bluetick hound dog. I. Clinical manifestations. Can. Vet. J. 15:303–8.

Fankhauser, R., H. Luginbuhl, and W. Hartley. 1963. Leukodystrophie vom typus krabbe beim hund. Schweiz. Arch. Tierheilkd. 105:198–207.

Fletcher, T. F., and H. J. Kurtz. 1972. Animal model for human disease: Globoid cell leukodystrophy in the dog. Am. J. Pathol. 66:375–78.

Fletcher, T. F., H. J. Kurtz, and D. Low. 1966. Globoid cell leukodystrophy (Krabbe type) in the dog. JAVMA 149:165–72.

Fletcher, T. F., D. G. Lee, and R. F. Hammer. 1971. Ultrastructural features of globoid cell leukodystrophy in the dog. Am. J. Vet. Res. 32:177–81.

Hirth, R. S., and S. W. Nielsen. 1967. A familial canine globoid cell leukodystrophy (Krabbe type). J. Small Anim. Pract. 8:569–75.

Hoerlein, B. F. 1971. Canine Neurology: Diagnosis and treatment, 2nd ed. Philadelphia, London, Toronto: W. B. Saunders.

Howell, J. McC., and A. C. Palmer. 1971. Globoid cell leukodystrophy in two dogs. J. Small Anim. Pract. 12:633–42.

Johnson, G. R., J. E. Oliver, and R. Selcer. 1975. Globoid cell leukodystrophy in a beagle. JAVMA 167:380–84.

Jortner, B., and A. Jonas. 1968. The neuropathology of globoid cell leukodystrophy in the dog. Acta Neuropathol. 10:171–82.

McGrath, J., H. Schutta, A. Yaseen, and S. Steinberg. 1969. A morphologic and biochemical study of canine globoid leukodystrophy. J. Neuropathol. Exp. Neurol. 28:171.

Suzuki, Y., J. Austin, D. Armstrong, K. Suzuki, J. Schlenker, and T. F. Fletcher. 1970. Studies in globoid leukodystrophy: Enzymatic and lipid findings in the canine form. Exper. Neurol. 19:65–75.

Zaki, F. A., and W. L. Kay. 1973. Globoid cell leukodystrophy in a miniature poodle. JAVMA 163:248–50.

SCOTTIE CRAMP

A condition exists in the Scottish terrier that results in intermittent spasticity or difficult locomotion following strenuous exercise or excitement. One may observe an arching of the back in the lumbar region, involving back and neck, or a stiff legged gait with the back legs overflexed and the front legs greatly abducted when walking. When running, the dog may hop with one or both legs held against the body. If activity continues, some dogs may become unable to walk and will assume a pillarlike stance. Dogs do not lose consciousness. If the dog is allowed to rest for a few minutes, the condition will correct itself. A great deal of variation is noted among dogs. The defect may be observed as early as 6 weeks of age and usually is fully developed before 1 year of age. The muscular hypertonicity appears to be the result of a central nervous system defect rather than a muscle defect.

Inheritance and Recommendation

Evidence suggests that Scottie cramp is inherited as an autosomal recessive.

Select against this trait as a recessive.

REFERENCES

Joshua, J. C. 1956. Scottie Cramp. Vet. Rec. 68:411–12.

Meyers, K. M., and W. M. Dickson. 1969. Indolealkylamines and hyperkinetic episodes in Scottish terrier dogs. Fed. Proc. 28:794.

Meyers, K. M., J. E. Lund, and J. T. Boyce. 1968. Muscular cramping of central nervous system origin in Scottish terrier dogs. Fed. Proc. 27:611.

Meyers, K. M., J. E. Lund, G. A. Padgett, and W. M. Dickson. 1969. Hyperkinetic episodes in Scottish terrier dogs. JAVMA 155:129-33.
Smythe, R. H. 1945. Recurrent tetany in the dog. Vet. Rec. 57:380.

STOCKARD'S PARALYSIS

A paralysis of the posterior extremities has been reported to occur in the Saint Bernard, Great Dane, bloodhound, and/or crosses between these breeds. Pups appear normal until they reach 11-14 weeks of age, at which time gradually or in some cases suddenly the pups are unable to move their hind legs. Some pups will be completely down and unable to rise or push with hind legs; some can walk with assistance. Pain is not expressed, and after a few days to a month pups may learn to walk, but with difficulty. Weakness and a faulty gait are noted. In milder cases and in older dogs, the legs appear somewhat stiffened and animals have a slightly narrowed and atrophied rump region.

Pathophysiology

The condition results from the death and/or destruction of certain motor and preganglionic sympathetic neurons in the lateral and anterior horns of the lumbar region of the spinal cord. Microglia accumulate and migrate along the axons of motor neurons and infiltrate the ventral roots of the lumbar region. The cells play an active role in the destruction and cleanup of dead neurons and axons but do not cause the death. Also noted in males is a chronic dilation of the vessels of the erectile tissue.

Inheritance and Recommendation

The condition appears to result from a certain combination of at least three dominant genes. For the trait to be expressed, at least one member of each of the three pairs must be present in the dominant state.

Avoid the breeding of closely related animals of affected pups and select against the dominant genes.

REFERENCE

Stockard, C. 1936. An hereditary lethal for localized motor and preganglionic neurones with a resulting paralysis in the dog. Am. J. Anat. 59:1-53.

SPINAL DYSRAPHISM (Syringomyelia)

Dysraphism is the improper union or fusion between two contiguous or similar structures, or the incomplete closure of the primary neural tube. Spinal dysraphism or syringomyelia has been observed in Weimaraners. The first signs of the defect appear at 4-6 weeks of age and are usually not progressive. As one would expect, there is a variability of clinical signs. Reportedly one always observes degrees of a symmetrical hopping hind-leg gait when walking and especially when running, as well as stances in which the dog assumes a crouching posture as though frightened. Frequently there is a unilateral abduction of one hind limb, and the dog may overextend the hind limbs when standing. Young dogs also may exhibit a depressed hind-paw position sense.

Clinical signs observed on occasion include scoliosis of the spine in the lower thoracic and anterior lumbar region, anomalies of hair growth in the dorsal neck region, a gutterlike depression of the chest, occasionally kinked tail, and some disproportion in length of limbs.

Pathophysiology

Structural abnormalities of the spinal cord include anomalies of the central canal such as hydromyelia with or without syringomyelia, the absence of or duplication of the central canal, and unusually shaped or eccentric central canal.

Anomalies of the ventral median fissure include variations in its size or its complete absence (dysraphic lesions). Syringomyelia includes small to large cavitations of the spinal cord. Gross defects were most frequent in the thoracic region (older animals) and some hydromyelia was found in newborn and young pups.

Inheritance and Recommendation

Data presented are not sufficient to make definite conclusions as to the type of gene action. However, the variation in phenotypic expression may suggest polygenetic or multigenetic action. According to one author's interpretation, the condition may result from a dominant gene with reduced penetrance.

Do not use affected animals or closely related animals in a breeding program if they are capable of reproducing. One could test as for a dominant trait. This should provide valuable information regardless of means of transmission.

REFERENCES

Confer, A. W., and B. C. Ward. 1972. Spinal dysraphism: A congenital myelodysplasia in the Weimaraner. JAVMA 160:1423–26.

Geib, L. W., and S. I. Bistner. 1967. Spinal cord dysraphism in the dog. JAVMA 150:618–20.

Kalter, H. 1968. Teratology of the central nervous system. Chicago and London: Univ. of Chicago Press.

McGrath, J. T. 1965. Spinal dysraphism in the dog with comments on syringomyelia. Pathol. Vet. 2(Suppl.):1–36.

CEREBELLAR CORTICAL AND EXTRAPYRAMIDAL NUCLEAR ABIOTROPHY

An inherited progressive disorder of function, represented by clinical signs of progressive cerebellar ataxia with spasticity, occurs in the Kerry blue terrier.

The defect is usually first observed in pups between the ages of 9 and 16 weeks. Initial signs include stiffness of the back legs and head tremors. Soon thereafter (2–3 weeks) the pups experience a further progressive abnormality in gait resulting in a mild basewide pelvic limb ataxia, with hypertonia represented by limited flexion of the hip, stifle, and tarsus during the protraction phase. Gait is dysmetric, but position sense is maintained. The thoracic limbs then become affected, the side-to-side head tremors continue, and intended head movements are exaggerated.

By 8–10 weeks after the initial signs of the condition are noticed, truncal ataxia is sufficient to make walking difficult. Head, trunk, and limb movements are disorganized. After about 20 weeks the dog is no longer able to stand, and skeletal muscle atrophy is evident. Proper response to postural tests is lost.

Pathophysiology

Lesions vary with the course of the disease. At first one finds progressive cerebellar cortical degeneration with loss of Purkinje's cells, followed by bilateral symmetric degeneration of the olivary nuclei and bilateral degeneration of the substantia nigra and caudate nucleus.

Inheritance and Recommendation

Autosomal recessive inheritance is proposed for this condition. Select against this trait as for any recessive.

REFERENCES

de Lahunta, A., and D. R. Averill. 1976. Hereditary cerebellar cortical and extrapyramidal nuclear abiotrophy in Kerry blue terriers. JAVMA 168:1119–24.
Mettler, F. A., and L. J. Goss. 1946. Canine chorea due to strio-cerebellar degeneration of unknown etiology. JAVMA 108:377–84.

MUSCLE FIBER DEFICIENCY

A rare but supposed inherited deficiency of type II muscle fibers has been reported in the Labrador retriever. Clinical signs included abnormal head and neck posture because of the inability of the pup to hold up its head following exercise, and a muscular weakness throughout the body.

The puppy's limbs were extended and it walked with stiff minor steps and a stiff forced hopping gait. Clinical signs disappeared with rest. The deficiency of muscle mass was sufficient to alter the dog's conformation. Stress due to cold, exercise, or excitement exaggerated the condition. The condition stabilized as the dog matured, and the older animal was stunted with less skeletal muscle mass. The condition was first noticed before the pup reached 6 months of age.

Histologic studies show a variation in fiber diameter and an increase in endomyseal and perimyseal connective tissue. Type I fibers predominate and the number of type II fibers is reduced. Marked creatinuria was found in the affected dogs. Serum CPK activity of affected dogs was lower than that of the controls.

Inheritance and Recommendation

The condition in the Labrador breed is rare. Pedigree studies suggest an inherited disorder, and the authors indicate that based on available data the disorder may be transmitted as an autosomal recessive.

Assuming the condition is recessive, a breeding program should be designed to eliminate the condition as for any other recessive gene.

REFERENCE

Kramer, J. W., G. A. Hegreberg, G. M. Bryan, K. Meyers, and R. L. Ott. 1976. A muscle disorder of Labrador retrievers characterized by deficiency of type II muscle fibers. JAVMA 169:817–20.

CHAPTER 7

Digestive System

CLEFT LIP AND PALATE

The palate is the partition dividing the oral and nasal cavities. It consists of the hard palate formed by bony plates and the soft palate which is basically muscle. A mucous membrane covers the palate. The closure process involves a complicated interaction of the bony plate, tongue resistance, mandible growth, and head growth.

Cleft palate is a condition observed in the dog in which the bony plates forming the roof of the mouth fail to properly close prior to birth. The cleft frequently terminates in a hairlip. Cleft palate occurs most frequently in the brachycephalic breeds such as the bulldog, Boston terrier, and boxer. The condition has been reported in many breeds, for example, toy poodle, Norwegian elkhound, Bernese mountain dog, beagle, cocker spaniel, Staffordshire terrier, dachshund, German shepherd, Shih Tzu, Chihuahua, Pekingese, bull mastiff, bull terrier, and collie. Although it is always recognized that *in utero* environmental conditions may be responsible for this trait, the increased incidence of cleft palate in certain breeds is strongly suggestive of a hereditary factor. Variation in the expression of this trait occurs, however, and it also accompanies other defects. Some pups that appear normal at birth may, upon nursing, aspirate milk in the nasal passages. In severe cases, the hard palate is divided into two separate halves, with a division in the center that communicates with the nasal chambers.

Inheritance and Recommendation

The mode of inheritance for cleft palate is not well defined and may differ among breeds. A simple dominant type of inheritance has been suggested for the Bernese mountain dog. Some authors feel that the condition for most breeds is recessive, but some data presented would also fit a dominant type of gene action. Simple dominant or recessive gene action might not fully explain all conditions, since cleft palate may be one of a series of anomalies and does vary in expression. This might strongly suggest multifactoral or polygenic control, and various environmental factors may be involved. Several distinct syndromes are recognized. It would appear that selection in certain breeds for a particular conformation has enhanced this trait, that is, the compression of the nasal cavity, pharynx, larynx, and surrounding tissue into an inadequate space.

Do not use for breeding those individuals having produced this defect or the close relatives of animals expressing this trait.

REFERENCES

Cooper, H. K., Jr., and G. W. Mattern. 1970. Genetic studies of cleft lip and palate in dogs (boxer breed): A preliminary report. Carnivore Genet. Newsletter No. 9, pp. 204–9.

Dreyer, C. J., and C. B. Preston. 1974. Classification of cleft lip and palate in animals. Cleft Palate J. 11:327–32.

Edmonds, L., R. W. Stewart, and L. Shelby. 1972. Cleft lip and palate in dogs (boxer breed): A preliminary report. Carnivore Genet. Newsletter No. 9, pp. 204–9.

_____. 1972. Cleft lip and palate in Boston terrier pups. Vet. Med. Small Anim. Clin., Nov. 1972, pp. 1219–22.

Fox, M. W. 1964. Thoracic congenital defects in the dog, specifically. Mod. Vet. Pract., pp. 45–70.

Fuller, J. L. 1954. Heredity and structural defects in dogs: Newer knowledge about dogs. Gaines Vet. Symp.

Gaines Dog Research Progress. Summer 1973. Cleft palate: The elusive anomaly.

Gardner, J. E., Jr. September 1954. Report of a survey on cleft palates in the English bulldog. Bull. Bulldog Club of New Jersey.

Hammer, D. L., and M. Socks. 1971. Surgical closure of cleft soft palate in a dog. JAVMA 158:342–45.

Horowitz, S. L., and H. B. Chase. 1970. A microform of cleft palate in the dog. J. Dent. Res. 49:892.

Jurkiewicz, M. J. 1964. A study of cleft lip and palate in dogs. Surgical Forum 15:457–58.

_____. 1964. Cleft lip and palate in dogs. Surg. Forum 15:457–58.

_____. 1965. A genetic study of cleft lip and palate in dogs. Surg. Forum 16:472–73.

Jurkiewicz, M. S., and D. L. Bryant. 1968. Cleft lip and palate in dogs: A progress report. Cleft Palate J. 5:30–36.

Marienfield, C. J., S. L. Silbery, R. W. Menges, W. T. Crawford, and H. T. Wright. 1967. Multispecies of congenital malformations in Missouri. Mo. Med. 64:230–33.

Setty, L. R. 1958. Cleft lip and palate in the dog. JAVMA 133:480.

ESOPHAGEAL ACHALASIA

Achalasia refers to the inability to relax. Esophageal achalasia (failure to open) means that the opening from the esophagus into the stomach does not relax sufficiently to allow the ingested food to enter the stomach. The result is the retention of food, the ballooning out of the esophagus, and persistent vomiting. Vomiting is apparently without strain. Vomiting of undigested food occurs within a few minutes to 2 hours after the dog has eaten, and the undigested bolus of food is covered with saliva and mucus. The inability to properly swallow the solid food causes weight loss, increased appetite, weakness, dehydration, and faulty bone mineralization as a secondary influence of poor nutrition. The condition usually does not fully express itself until the pup is weaned and begins to consume solid food. Some breeders have reported a gurgling sound as affected pups nurse.

The condition has been reported in many breeds, including the German shepherd, greyhound, wirehaired fox terrier, Rhodesian Ridgeback, schnauzer, dachshund, Dalmatian, springer spaniel, cocker spaniel, boxer, Labrador retriever, and Boston terrier.

Pathophysiology

The basic cause of esophageal achalasia is unknown. In the human, the absence or reduction of certain nerve cells, i.e., enteric neurons or ganglion cells, seems to be a factor. This has not been well demonstrated in the dog. However, some literature supports an imbalance of sympathetic-parasympathetic innervation of the esophagus, which results in failure of the terminal portion of the esophagus to relax after swallowing, as a possible cause. The disease includes a disturbance in esophageal mobility as well as increased resistance at the cardia.

Inheritance and Recommendation

Early reports suggested sex linkage to be involved in esophageal achalasia, but subsequent information has not verified this. Also suggested by some reports was a recessive condition. More recently, at least in wirehaired fox terriers and perhaps other breeds, an autosomal dominant was given as the mode of transmission.

In view of the most recent evidence, consider the condition as a dominant and breed accordingly. Consider also, however, that this might be transmitted differently in different breeds.

REFERENCES

Baronti, A. C. 1950. Congenital esophageal dilatation in a cocker puppy. North Am. Vet. 31:666–67.
Brasmer, T. H. 1953. Congenital esophageal dilatation. North Am. Vet. 34:36–38.
Breshears, D. E. 1965. Esophageal dilatation in six-week-old male German shepherd pups. Vet. Med. Small Anim. Clin. 60:1034–36.
Carlson, W. D., and W. V. Lumb. 1958. Esophageal invagination of the stomach in a dog. Mod. Vet. Pract. 39(5):65.
Clifford, D. H., and F. Gyorkey. 1967. Myenteric ganglial cells in dogs with and without achalasia of the esophagus. JAVMA 150:205–11.

Clifford, D. H., E. D. Waddell, D. R. Patterson, C. F. Wilson, and H. L. Thompson. 1972. Management of esophageal achalasia in miniature schnauzers. JAVMA 161:1012-21.

Diamant, N., M. Szczepanski, and H. Mui. 1973. Manometric characteristics of idiopathic megaesophagus in the dog: An unsuitable animal model for achalasia in man. Gastroenterology 65:216-23.

Earlam, R. J., P. E. Zollman, and F. H. Ellis, Jr. 1967. Congenital oesophageal achalasia in the dog. Thorax 22:466-72.

Fitts, R. H. 1948. Dilatation of the esophagus in a cocker spaniel. JAVMA 112:343-44.

Hofmeyer, C. F. B. 1955. Cardioplasty for achalasia in the dog. Vet. Med. 51:115-18.

Knecht, C. D., and J. A. Eaddy. 1959. Canine esophageal achalasia corrected by retrograde dilatation: A case report. JAVMA 135:554-55.

Lacroix, J. V. 1940. Cardiospasm in a puppy. North Am. Vet. 21:673-75.

_____. 1949. Congenital dilatation of the esophagus. North Am. Vet. 30:29-30.

Morgan, J. P., and W. V. Lumb. 1964. Achalasia of the esophagus in the dog. JAVMA 144:722-26.

Spy, G. M. 1963. Megaloesophagus in a litter of greyhounds. Vet. Rec. 75:853-55.

Stock, W. F., J. D. Thompson, and R. Suyama. 1957. Achalasia of the esophagus with megaesophagus in a dog. JAVMA 131:225-26.

Strating, A., and D. H. Clifford. 1966. Canine achalasia with special reference to heredity. Southwest. Vet. 19:135-37.

INTESTINAL LYMPHANGIECTASIA

A diarrheal syndrome characterized by malabsorption, a protein-losing enteropathy (disease of the intestine), and hypergammaglobulinemia (excess gamma globulin in the blood) has been observed in both male and female basenji pups. Pedigree studies strongly suggest that an autosomal recessive gene is responsible for the condition. A protein-losing enteropathy that appears to have a genetic basis has also been found for the Lunderhund breed of dog.

Clinical signs include depression, an unresponsive light brown to yellowish diarrhea with occasional blood, fever, vomiting, neurologic signs that may include the twitching of facial muscles, incoordination, seizures and paresis (paralysis), gradual deterioration, and weight loss.

Stressors such as vaccination may initiate the condition.

Pathophysiology

During the normal process of protein breakdown, amino acids are lost into the intestine but are normally reabsorbed. In this condition they are lost.

A histopathologic diagnosis of intestinal lymphangiectasia was made in two of four cases studied. The other two of the four cases had a diffuse lymphocytic-plasmacytic enteritis.

Inheritance and Recommendation

As indicated above, the condition is probably the result of an autosomal recessive gene.

Select against this trait as for any recessive. Breed test animals related to affected dogs.

REFERENCES

Campbell, R. S. F., D. Brobst, and G. Bisgard. 1968. Intestinal lymphangiectasia in a dog. JAVMA 153:1050–54.
Fox, I. W., W. G. Hoag, and J. Strout. 1965. Breed susceptibility, pathogenicity, and epidemiology of endemic coliform enteritis in the dog. Lab. Anim. Care 15(3):194–200.

LIVER DISEASE

A chronic progressive hepatitis or liver disease associated with increased liver copper concentrations has been reported in Bedlington terriers. The condition appears to be similar to Wilson's disease in humans. A genetic base is indicated since the disease is found primarily in the Bedlington.

Clinical signs are varied. All dogs do not respond similarly. Reports show that stress may initiate the condition in young adult dogs. Clinical signs include depression, lethargy, lack of appetite (anorexia), and vomiting. The dog may exhibit a jaundice condition (yellowing of mucous membranes). Death often occurs within 48–72 hours after the onset of initial symptoms. If the dog survives the initial attack, it may show no further clinical signs or in some cases exhibit recurring attacks.

Other dogs, usually older dogs, may show more chronic and less severe signs. In addition to the above-mentioned clinical symptoms, these older dogs may experience weight loss and ascites (accumulation of fluid in the body cavity) late in the course of the disease. Anemia is also common.

In still other dogs, usually young individuals, no clinical signs are observed (asymptomatic) and the condition can be detected only by biochemical tests. These tests can diagnose the problem as early as 3 months of age.

Pathophysiology

The condition appears to result from a chronic progressive hepatitis.

It is believed that massive hepatocellular necrosis occurs, resulting in a rapid release of intracellular copper into the blood. The elevated blood copper concentrations damage the membranes of the red blood cell, causing it to rupture.

A copper-related metabolic defect may be involved.

Inheritance and Recommendation

Since the condition is found for the most part only in the Bedlington, this would suggest an inherited condition. The mode of inheritance is yet to be determined.

Without further information on the mode of inheritance involved, one cannot make detailed recommendations. However, test all breeding stock, and avoid the use of affected animals and close relatives to such animals if possible.

REFERENCES

Hardy, R. M., and J. B. Stevens. 1977. Chronic progressive hepatitis in Bedlington terriers (Bedlington liver disease). Current Veterinary Therapy. VI. Philadelphia, London, Toronto: W. B. Saunders, pp. 995–98.

Hardy, R. M., J. B. Stevens, and C. M. Stowe. 1975. Chronic progressive hepatitis in Bedlington terriers associated with elevated liver copper concentrations. Minn. Vet. 15(6):13–24.

CHAPTER 8

Endocrine and Metabolic Systems

PITUITARY DWARFISM

An inherited pituitary dwarfism has been reported in various breeds but occurs most frequently in the German shepherd.

Pups appear normal at birth, and clinical signs are not obvious for the first 1 or 2 months of the pups' lives. In addition to growth retardation, an alteration in hair coat is observed.

The adult dog will be extremely small but well proportioned, with partial puppylike hair coat (wooly, irregular fur), accompanied by a symmetrical hair loss. In one case the dog in question became obese. The skin was thin and fragile.

Pathophysiology

Some reports consider cystic hypofunctioning pituitary gland as the cause. Low somatomedin activity was found in the plasma of four related German shepherd dwarf dogs. Somatomedin is a growth-promoting hormonelike substance found in plasma and controlled by the growth hormone. The pituitary gland may be almost completely replaced by multiceptic remnants of Rathke's cleft. These are filled with mucin and lined by cuboidal and ciliated columnar epithelium containing numerous goblet cells.

Inheritance and Recommendation

The syndrome might be regarded as a threshold character based on polygenic inheritance. However, the data given also could fit a simple autosomal recessive pattern. The authors of some articles appear to favor recessive inheritance. Assumed heterozygous relatives of affected dogs appear to be intermediate for somatomedin.

Select against this gene by not using breeding stock whose offspring and close relatives show this trait. When a definite pattern of inheritance is established, other recommendations could be made.

REFERENCES

Andersen, R., P. Willeberg, and P. G. Rasmussen. 1974. Pituitary dwarfism in German shepherd dogs: Genetic investigations. Nord. Vet. Med. 26:692–701.

Baker, E. 1955. Congenital hypoplasia of the pituitary and pancreas glands in the dog. JAVMA 126:468–69.

Jensen, E. C. 1959. Hypopituitarism associated with cystic Rathke's cleft in a dog. JAVMA 135:572–75.

Muller, G. H., and S. R. Jones. 1973. Pituitary dwarfism and alopecia in a German shepherd with a cystic Rathke's cleft. JAAHA 9:567–72.

Willeberg, P., K. W. Kastrup, and E. Andersen. 1975. Pituitary dwarfism in German shepherd dogs: Studies on somatomedin activity. Nord. Vet. Med. 27:448–54.

CHAPTER 9

Urogenital System

CRYPTORCHIDISM

In mammalian species one observes males in which the testes do not descend into the scrotum. These animals are referred to as cryptorchids (*kryptos,* concealed, and *orchis,* testes). If both testicles are retained, the animal is a bilateral cryptorchid. If only one testicle fails to descend into the scrotum, the animal is a unilateral cryptorchid. The unilateral cryptorchid is often incorrectly referred to as a monorchid. The term monorchid means that the animal has only one testicle and this of course is not true, since the dog has two testicles, but only one has descended.

Some reports estimate the number of cryptorchid dogs to be between 0.05% and 0.1%. Several recent reports suggest a much higher incidence. In one small animal practice, 12.9% of 1,494 male dogs examined were classified as cryptorchids. Of these 1,494 dogs, 30 of those examined were under 6 months of age at the time of the initial examination and testicular descent occurred later. Twenty-seven other cryptorchid dogs under 6 months of age at the time of the initial examination were not rechecked. When these 57 dogs were removed from consideration, the percentage was 9.2. This percentage is comparable to other recent reports. One expects cryptorchidism to be much higher in certain strains and families of dogs.

Cryptorchidism is a developmental defect. The cryptorchid condition may be completely abdominal, which implies that the testis, epididymis, etc., are all within the body cavity, or this condition may be incompletely abdominal, which suggests that only a portion of the testis or its appendages are retained in the abdominal cavity or inguinal canal. Inguinal cryptorchidism exists when the testes are in the inguinal canal.

The descent of the testis of the dog may be somewhat slower than for other species. While the testes of the pup may be present in the scrotum near the time of birth, it is not uncommon for the testes to be retained much longer. The majority of practitioners feel that the testicles should be palpable by 6–8 weeks of age. Most feel that a definite diagnosis should not be made until the dog is 6–12 months of age.

Pathophysiology

The bilateral cryptorchid animal is sterile, and spermatogenesis is inhibited because of a high testicular temperature. Elevated temperatures for a short period of time, under experimental conditions, result in disarrangement of the germinal epithelium, folding of the basement membrane, and infiltration of the Sertoli cells with fat. These conditions are reversible unless the animal is exposed to elevated temperatures for prolonged periods of time as would be the case for cryptorchids. Apparently the degeneration of tissue is due to a lack of sufficient oxygen or substrate.

In the unilateral cryptorchid, spermatogenesis appears normal in the testicle observed in the scrotal sac but is abnormal or completely lacking in the testicle retained within the body cavity.

The production of the male hormone, testosterone, by the interstitial Leydig cells continues in the undescended testes. This is true for both the bilateral and unilateral cryptorchid. Testosterone production in retained testicles may be somewhat lower than normal in certain species.

Inheritance and Recommendation

Evidence suggests that some cases of cryptorchidism are genetic in origin. Species differences in the mode of inheritance may exist. For the dog, most research reports suggest that the cryptorchid condition is the result of a sex-limited autosomal recessive gene. Some reports indicate that cryptorchidism is not controlled by a single gene but possibly by two gene pairs. The descent of each testicle would be controlled by one gene pair. This theory would allow nine different genotypes, five of which would allow for some form of cryptorchidism to be expressed. Penetrance may also be low for this characteristic.

The majority of veterinary practitioners have found little success in trying to correct the cryptorchid condition with hormone therapy. Unilateral or bilateral cryptorchids should not be used for breeding. If possible avoid the use of dogs that have sired cryptorchids.

REFERENCES

Ashdown, R. R. 1963. Diagnosis of cryptorchidism in young dogs: A review of the problem. J. Small Anim. Pract. 4(4):261–63.

Bishop, M. W. H. 1972. Genetically determined abnormalities of the reproductive system. J. Reprod. Fertil. Suppl. 15:51–78.

British Veterinary Association. 1955. Cryptorchidism in the dog. Vet. Rec. 67:472-74.
Brodey, R. S., and J. S. Reif. 1969. Relationship between canine testicular neoplasia and cryptorchidism. JAVMA 154:1358.
Dunn, M. L., W. J. Foster, and K. M. Goddard. 1968. Incidence of cryptorchidism. JAAHA 4:180.
Gaines Dog Research Report. Fall 1971. Cryptorchidism: The "not" entire dog, p. 7.
Lindo, D. E., and H. H. Grenn. 1969. Case report: Bilateral Sertoli cell tumor in a canine cryptorchid with accompanying pathological lesions. Can. Vet. J. 10:145-47.
Marsboom, R., J. Spruyt, and C. H. Van Ravestyn. 1971. Incidence of congenital abnormalities in a beagle colony. Lab. Anim. 5:41-48.
Panel Report. 1971. Cryptorchidism. Mod. Vet. Pract. 52(8):41-46.
Pullig, T. 1953. Cryptorchidism in cocker spaniels. J. Hered. 44:250-64.
Reif, J. S., and R. S. Brodey. 1969. The relationship between cryptorchidism and canine testicular neoplasia. JAVMA 155:2005-10.
Technical Development Committee Report. 1954. Cryptorchidism with special references to the condition in the dog. Vet. Rec. 66:482-83.
Turner, T. 1970. Torsion of the retained testicle in the dog. J. Small Anim. Pract. 11:436.
Willis, M. B. 1960. Inheritance of cryptorchidism. J. Anim. Health Trust 21-25.
———. 1963. Abnormalities and defects in pedigree dogs. V. Cryptorchidism. J. Small Anim. Pract. 4:469-74.

INTERSEXUALITY (HERMAPHRODITISM, PSEUDOHERMAPHRODITISM)

Hermaphroditism (intersexuality) refers to an animal in which varying degrees of internal and external organs of both sexes are found. The condition is usually classified according to the presence of ovarian or testicular tissue. If a dog contains both ovaries and testes, the animal would be classified as a true hermaphrodite. A pseudohermaphrodite may be either male or female. The male pseudohermaphrodites would have testes and either or both male and female internal and external secondary sex organs. Female pseudohermaphrodites would have ovaries with either or both male and female internal and external secondary sex organs. Therefore, classification of intersexuality is based on the gonads present and not on the genetic sex of the dog. Variations exist in the completeness of the reproductive tracts of both sexes within one individual and as to the chromosome (XX, XY) genotype in relation to gonadal tissue and genitalia.

Intersexuality is relatively rare in the dog but has been reported for several breeds.

Pathophysiology

No good single explanation seems to fit all cases. In some dogs, but not all, a genetic base seems likely. One theory suggested was that in some genetic males and females Mullerian derivatives remain, regardless of gonadal sex. The persistence of the Wolffian derivatives is correlated with the extent of gonad development as testes. It was suggested that the X chromosome contains homologous male-determining genes that can be either repressed or activated. Activation is normally effected by the Y chromosome in the male complement, but in the abnormal female genotype it can also be brought about by aberrant autosomal influence. Apparently the Mullerian system of ducts is not suppressed as it would normally be in the presence of a testes. Suppression is mediated by the testicular hormone. It could be that the testicles produce the proper hormone, but the tissue of the ducts fails to respond properly and remains inactive or persists. Also the genes controlling testicular development, which should be inactive in the normal XX individual, may be functional to a considerable degree but not completely functional as in the normal animal. Their activity is sufficient, however, to allow development of a normal-appearing structure (but sterile).

The male hormone production is sufficient to allow various degrees of development of masculinity, but it is suggested that the activation of genes controlling testes development is incomplete so the hormone that supresses the Mullerian system is not produced.

Inheritance and Recommendation

Indications are that intersexuality in some dogs is inherited. This is suggested since the condition has occurred when all affected dogs had a common ancestor and the intersexuality was reported more often in certain breeds. A mode of gene action or detailed recommendations on the control of this defect cannot be given with the limited data available, but some authors suggest an autosomal recessive gene. Other reports, however, have suggested a sex-linked recessive and some a dominant with incomplete penetrance.

REFERENCES

Bishop, M. W. H. 1972. Genetically determined abnormalities of the reproductive system. J. Reprod. Fertil. Suppl. 15:51.

Brodey, R. S., J. D. Martin, and D. G. Lee. 1954. Male pseudohermaphroditism in a toy terrier. JAVMA 125:368.

Brown, R. D., M. C. Swanton, and K. M. Brinkhous. 1963. Canine hemophilia and male pseudohermaphroditism: Cytogenetic studies. Lab. Invest. 12:961.

Brown, T. T., J. D. Burek, and K. McEntee. 1976. Male pseudohermaphroditism, cryptorchidism, and Sertoli cell neoplasia in three miniature schnauzers. JAVMA 169:821.

Dain, A. R. 1974. Intersexuality in a cocker spaniel dog. J. Reprod. Fertil. 39:365.

Edols, J. H., and G. J. Allan. 1968. A case of male pseudohermaphroditism in a cocker spaniel. Aust. Vet. J. 44:287.

Hare, W. C. D. 1976. Intersexuality in dogs. Can. Vet. J. 17:7.

Hare, W. C. D., R. A. McFeely, and D. F. Kelly. 1974. Familial 78 XX male pseudohermaphroditism in three dogs. J. Reprod. Fertil. 36:207.

McFeely, R. A., and J. D. Biggers. 1965. A rare case of female pseudohermaphroditism in the dog. Vet. Rec. 77:696–98.

Schneck, G. W. 1975. Hermaphroditism in a Shetland sheepdog. Vet. Rec. 96:323.

Schultz, M. G. 1962. Male pseudohermaphroditism diagnosed with aid of sechromatin technique. JAVMA 140:241.

Stewart, R. W., R. W. Menges, L. A. Selby, J. D. Rhoades, and D. B. Crenshaw. 1962. Canine intersexuality in a pug breeding kennel. Cornell Vet. 62(3):464.

RENAL CORTICAL HYPOPLASIA

Renal cortical hypoplasia is a reduced amount of renal cortical (outer zone of the kidney) tissue. The condition has been found in the cocker spaniel, German shepherd, dachshund, Doberman pinscher, Norwegian elkhound, and Lhasa Apso. The defect is usually first manifested between 3 months and 3 years of age, with a large percentage of the cases occurring at approximately 12 months of age. Clinical signs are those of a chronic, progressive renal disease. These include polyuria and polydipsia (excessive urination and thirst), intermittent anorexia, vomiting, occasional diarrhea, and weight loss. Glucosuria and proteinuria (glucose and protein in urine) may be present. If uremia occurs before the pup has completed its growth, dwarfing may result. Some tenderness at the jaws when eating has been observed; varying degrees of severity will be noted among individuals.

Pathophysiology

A marked reduction in the number of glomeruli in the renal cortex is observed and many glomerular tufts are atrophic. There are generalized nephrosclerosis and nephrocalcinosis and a marked dilation of the tubules without active inflammatory reaction.

Secondary hyperparathyroidism occurs as a result of calcium and phosphorous imbalances. The decreased number of functional nephrons leads to phosphorous retention and in turn hypocalcemia. Excess parathyroid hormone is produced, but additional hormone is required. The parathyroid gland was found to have chief cell hyperplasia with many acinar cellular arrangements. A generalized osteodystrophia fibrosa occurs with the more severe lesions in the mandible.

Inheritance and Recommendation

Renal cortical hypoplasia is probably inherited as a recessive trait.

Select against the trait as against any recessive.

REFERENCES

Finco, D. R. 1974. Congenital and inherited renal diseases. In Current Veterinary Therapy, edited by R. W. Kirk. Philadelphia, London, Toronto: W. B. Saunders.

Kaufman, C. F., R. F. Soirez, and J. P. Tasker. 1969. Renal hypoplasia with secondary hyperparathyroidism in the dog. JAVMA 155:1679–85.

Krook, L. 1957. The pathology of renal cortical hypoplasia in the dog. Nord. Vet. Med. 9:161–76.

Persson, F., S. Persson, and A. Asheim. 1961. Renal cortical hypoplasia in dogs: A clinical study on uremia and secondary hyperparathyroidism. Acta Vet. Scand. 2:68–84.

POLYCYSTIC KIDNEY

Polycystic mononephrosis has been reported in the beagle. Cystic degeneration of the kidney results in renal failure, uremia, and death. Upon examination, adult dogs that died of chronic interstitial nephritis had only one kidney. Polycystic lesions were superimposed on lesions resulting from chronic interstitial nephritis. The cystic lesions could have been attributed to sequential change due to chronic interstitial nephritis, but the apparent susceptibility to *Pseudomonas* infection suggested a congenital defect in the remaining kidney. Neonate pups were also found to have one kidney. Histologic examination revealed polycystic lesions within the cortex and medulla of the kidney.

Inheritance and Recommendation

Based on limited information, the defect is believed to be transmitted as a recessive.

Select against this condition as one would do for any other recessive.

REFERENCES

Fox, M. W. 1964. Inherited polycystic mononephrosis in the dog. J. Hered. 55:29–30.
McQueen, S. D., A. C. Directo, and B. F. Llorico. 1975. Bilateral congenital polycystic kidneys. Vet. Med. Small Anim. Clin. 70:1167–71.

URIC ACID EXCRETION

In most mammals (including dogs) metabolic degradation of purines passes through a uric acid stage to yield allantoin. The Dalmatian dog is an exception, and as in primates, it excretes uric acid in its urine. The high uric acid is a unique characteristic of this breed. There are no obvious clinical signs and the defect may be of no great clinical significance. One report suggested, however, that the increased amounts of uric acid excretion may result in a predisposition for renal calculi. It was pointed out that clinically the Dalmatian was not reported to have kidney stones in excess of other breeds, but the majority of kidneys examined from Dalmatians contained stones.

Pathophysiology

The excessive urinary uric acid excretion characteristic of the Dalmatian results from a genetically determined defect in proximal tubular reabsorption of filtered urate. A peculiarity of purine metabolism is believed to be an absence of tubular resorption of uric acid, but further investigations also showed that under some conditions the usual net resorption of uric acid can be replaced by a net secretion (also in the proximal tubule). In addition, it is believed that a defect is involved in the access of uric acid to the interior of various cells (kidney, liver, erythrocytes) because of a lack of mediated transport systems in erythrocytes or other cells. Other work has shown a probable deficiency of hepatic uricase as well. Liver uricase levels appear normal, but a functional deficiency in hepatic uricase activity appears to exist.

Inheritance and Recommendation

The condition results from an autosomal recessive.

Uric acid excretion exists in almost all if not all Dalmatians, so it would be difficult to remove; however, it is not necessarily detrimental and should be of no real concern.

REFERENCES

Duncan, H., K. G. Wakin, and L. E. Ward. 1961. The effects of intravenous administration of uric acid on its concentration in plasma and urine of Dalmatian and non-Dalmatian dogs. J. Lab. Clin. Med. 58:876-83.

Friedman, M., and S. O. Byers. 1948. Effect of sodium salicylate upon the uric acid clearance of the Dalmatian dog. Am. J. Physiol. 154:167-73.

_____. 1948. Observations concerning the causes of the excess excretion of uric acid in the Dalmatian dog. J. Biol. Chem. 175:727-35.

Harvey, A. M., and H. N. Christensen. 1964. Uric acid transport system: Apparent absence in erythrocytes of the Dalmatian coach hound. Science 145:826-27.

Keeler, C. F. 1940. The inheritance of predisposition to renal calculi in the Dalmatian. JAVMA 96:507-10.

Kessler, R. H., K. Hierholzer, and R. S. Gurd. 1959. Localization of urate transport in the nephron of mongrel and Dalmatian dog kidney. Am. J. Physiol. 197:601-83.

Miller, G. E., L. S. Danzig, and J. H. Talbott. 1951. Urinary excretion of uric acid in the Dalmatian and non-Dalmatian dogs following administration of drodrast, sodium salicylate, and a mercurial diuretic. Am. J. Physiol. 164:155-58.

Trimble, H. D., and C. E. Keeler. 1938. The inheritance of high uric acid excretion in dogs. J. Hered. 19:280-89.

Ts'Ai-Fan Yu, et al. 1971. Low uricase activity in Dalmatian dogs simulated in mongrels given uronic acid. Am. J. Physiol. 220:973-79.

Yu, T. F., L. Berger, and A. B. Gutman. 1966. Defective conversion of uric acid to allantoin in the Dalmatian dog. Arthritis Rheum. 9:552 (abst.).

Yu, T. F., L. Berger, S. Kupper, and A. B. Gutman. 1960. Tubular secretion of urate in the dog. Am. J. Physiol. 199:1199-1204.

CHAPTER 10

Skin

ATOPIC DERMATITIS

Certain dogs appear to have a predisposition to develop clinical signs of seasonal hypersensitivity subject to hereditary influences and resulting from pollens, etc. A reaginic antibody is the causative factor. Most atopic dogs are multisensitive. Variation is noted as to when clinical signs appear, but for most atopic dogs it is between the first and third years of life. Clinical signs are seasonal, but since many atopic dogs are multisensitive, the duration of clinical signs may extend over several months. The dog rubs or scratches its face, particularly the eyes and nose. The most prominent clinical signs are self-inflicted trauma from rubbing or scratching. Itching may be generalized and involve the axilla (armpit beneath the foreleg) and the digits, or it may be universal. Respiratory signs do not usually appear under natural conditions. Urticaria (hives) is not often observed.

In some studies, but not all, a few more cases have been observed in the female, but the condition definitely is found in both sexes. Certain breeds such as wirehaired terriers and Dalmatians are more subject to the condition than are other breeds; yet hypersensitivity to certain pollens occurs in some dogs of most breeds.

Pathophysiology

The basic defect in atopy is the ability of the affected individual to produce a unique antibody referred to as the reaginic antibody. Among other unusual qualities or characteristics is the ability of the reagin to fix to tissue and damage the local tissue.

Inheritance and Recommendation

The condition apparently has a familial or hereditary base as evidenced by its breed predilection and by family histories of affected dogs. Also the hereditary nature of the atopic dog has been demonstrated by breeding experiments. The exact mode of inheritance is not stated, but in one study in which both the sire and dam were atopic, the entire litter produced was atopic. In other matings where only one parent was atopic, a varying number of the pups were atopic.

Clinical signs are somewhat latent, so many animals may be used for breeding before the owner is aware of the condition. One must look at close relatives of dogs concerned and avoid the use of these relatives and affected dogs in a breeding program.

REFERENCES

Patterson, R. 1960. Investigations of spontaneous hypersensitivity of the dog. J. Allergy 31:351–63.
Patterson, R., J. J. Pruzansky, and W. W. Y. Chang. 1963. Spontaneous canine hypersensitivity to ragweed characterization of the serum factor transferring skin, bronchial and anaphylactic sensitivity. J. Immunol. 90:35–42.
Patterson, R., J. I. Tennenbaum, J. J. Pruzansky, and V. L. Nelson. 1965. Canine antiragweed serum: Demonstration of "blocking" activity by in vivo and in vitro techniques. J. Allergy 36:138–46.
Schwartzman, R. M. 1968. Clinical manifestations and treatment of atopy in the dog. Vet. Med. Small Anim. Clin. pp. 1131 36.
Schwartzman, R. M., and J. H. Rockey. 1967. Atopy in the dog. Arch. Dermatol. 96:418–22.
Schwartzman, R. M., J. H. Rockey, and R. E. Halliwell. 1971. Canine reaginic antibody: Characterization of the spontaneous anti-ragweed and induced anti-dinitrophenyl reaginic antibodies of the atopic dog. Clin. Exp. Immunol. 9:549–69.
Wittich, F. W. 1940. Spontaneous allergy (atopy) in the lower animal: Seasonal hay fever (fall type) in a dog. J. Allergy 12:247–51.

CUTANEOUS ASTHENIA (SKIN WEAKNESS)

Cutaneous asthenia is an inherited skin disorder reported in the springer spaniel, beagle, Manchester terrier, Welsh corgi and in mongrels. Clinical signs in dogs include fragility of skin and peripheral blood vessels, hyperextensibility, and laxity of the skin. The most pronounced clinical sign is the fragility of the skin. Lacerations are produced easily, with resultant large, gaping wounds but practically no hemorrhage. The skin of such animals has wide, pliable, thin scars. Minimal connective tissue deposition is observed in the scar tissue. Subcutaneous hematomas may develop at sites of injury. Folds and widening of the nasal bridge have been observed in affected dogs. Reports indicate that the skin over the entire body is loose, and the laxity is best observed on the legs. The skin has a moist, blanched appearance and is velvety in texture. The dermis feels thinner than normal and hair shafts form an acute angle with the epidermal surface and are visible through the overlying epidermis.

In the dog, involved extracutaneous tissues include mesentery, intestinal wall, aorta, and muscle attachments.

Pathophysiology

The basic defect is unknown. The most severe alteration involves the collagenous tissues. The dermis appears thin, with a lack of uniformity in size and orientation of the collagen bundles. Many collagen bundles are fragmented, shortened, and occasionally swollen. In some areas, the dermis has a myxomatous appearance, with ground substance and fine fibrillar elements predominating.

Inheritance and Recommendation

Cutaneous asthenia in dogs is genetically transmitted. It is a collagen abnormality inherited as an autosomal dominant trait with complete penetrance.

Remove animals showing the trait from the breeding program.

REFERENCES

Brown, M. A. 1947. Generalized acute cutaneous asthenia in a dog. J. Am. Vet. Med. Assoc. 110:234-35.

Loehning, M. A. 1971. Suspected Ehlers-Danlos syndrome in the dog. Vet. Rec. 89:638-41.

Hegreberg, G. A. 1975. Animal model of human disease: Ehlers-Danlos syndrome. Am. J. Pathol. 79:383–86.

Hegreberg, G. A., G. A. Padgett, J. B. Henson, and R. L. Ott. 1966. Cutaneous asthenia in dogs. Proc. 16th Gaines Vet. Symp. 1–4.

Hegreberg, G. A., G. A. Padgett, J. R. Gorham, and J. B. Henson. 1969. A connective tissue disease in dogs and mink resembling the Ehlers-Danlos syndrome of man. J. Hered. 60:249–54.

Hegreberg, G. A., G. A. Padgett, R. L. Ott, and J. B. Henson. 1970. A heritable connective tissue disease of dogs and mink resembling Ehlers-Danlos syndrome of man. I. Clinical changes and skin tensile strength properties. J. Invest. Dermatol. 54:377–80.

Hegreberg, G. A., G. A. Padgett, and J. B. Henson. 1970. A heritable connective tissue disease of dogs and mink resembling the Ehlers-Danlos syndrome of man. III. Histopathologic changes of the skin. Arch. Pathol. 90:159–66.

Keep, J. M. 1969. Cutes hyperelastica in a dog. Aust. Vet. J. 45:593.

Wall, R. D. 1947. Congenital defect of the skin. North Am. Vet. 28:166–68.

DERMOID SINUS

The Rhodesian Ridgeback is subject to a condition known as dermoid sinus.

A distinguishing characteristic found in some Rhodesian Ridgebacks and Ridgeback crosses is a ridge of hair on the back growing the opposite direction to other body hair. The dermoid sinus or "middorsal" cyst is found midline from a short distance behind the head to just before the beginning of the ridge, or beyond the end of the ridge to the rest of the tail.

It is most frequently found over the cervical vertebrae and to a lesser extent over the sacrococcygeal region. No cases of sinus involving the ridge have been reported. The sinuses may be single or up to eight in number. Those in the sacral area may be up to three in number. The dermoid sinuses do not cause symptoms unless they become infected. They are congenital and can be felt as thin cords, 1-5 mm in diameter, running between the skin and spine to the dura mater in the coccygeal region or the spinous process of the cervical vertebrae. The sinuses form a small external opening and the hair around the opening is concentrated in a tuft. These cords connect the skin and the dorsal spinous ligament but are not in communication with the dura mater in the neck or thoracic region, even though the dura may be involved in the sacral sinuses.

Pathophysiology

The sinus (long, thick-walled tubes with multiple outpouchings) is composed of fibrous tissue lined with squamous stratified epithelium. The surrounding connective tissue contains hair follicles that open through the lining epithelium. The hair shafts project into the lumen. Sebaceous glands are connected to these follicles and sweat glands are placed more peripherally.

In some dermoid sinuses the epithelium ends a short distance below the external skin. In others it ends near the point of attachment to the supraspinous ligament. The sinus tubes are single.

The condition results from incomplete separation (dehiscence) between the skin and spinal cord of the neural tube in early embryonic life.

Inheritance and Recommendation

The genetic transmission of the defect has not been clarified; several theories have been suggested. The condition occurs in puppies from sinus-free stock and in individuals without ridges. It may occur in crossbred dogs that do not resemble the Ridgeback and in dogs without a vestige of a ridge. Some authors suggest dominance with incomplete penetrance; one author suggests a recessive trait. A complex of genes (polygenic) may be involved and most Ridgebacks probably carry some of the factors.

Until further clarification of the mode of inheritance is made, one cannot make specific recommendations. However, one should select carefully and avoid use of affected animals if possible.

REFERENCES

Hofmeyer, C. F. B. 1963. Dermoid sinus in the Ridgeback dog. J. Small Anim. Pract. Suppl. 4:5–8.

Hyman, S. D. 1974. Letter to the editor. Can. Vet. J. 15:230.

Lord, L. H., A. J. Cawley, and J. Giliay. 1957. Mid-dorsal dermoid sinuses in Rhodesian Ridgeback dogs: A case report. JAVMA 131:515–18.

Mann, G. E., and J. Stratton. 1966. Dermoid sinus in the Rhodesian Ridgeback. J. Small Anim. Pract. 7:631–42.

Ross, G. R., and C. R. Howlett. 1974. Dermoid sinus in the Rhodesian Ridgeback in Australia. Aust. Vet. Pract. 4:173–81.

Steyn, H. P., J. Quinlan, and C. Jackson. 1939. A skin condition seen in Rhodesian Ridgeback dogs: Report of two cases. J. S. Afr. Vet. Med. Assoc. 10:170–74.

CHAPTER 11

Other Structures

DIAPHRAGMATIC HERNIA

In diaphragmatic hernia the tissues do not unite in the normal way to form the sheetlike diaphragm. The herniation is often located cranial to the right lobe of the liver and is usually small. Most diaphragmatic hernias are not considered to be inherited. Congenital diaphragmatic hernias of possible hereditary origin have been reported. Individual pups in the study were crossbred Labrador retrievers–American foxhounds. In this study only the sternal diaphragm and portions of the costal diaphragm had developed.

Faces of thick, blunt, diaphragmatic muscle extended bilaterally from the sternal segment to approximately the level of the right and left costochondral junctions. The tendinous center, most of the lateral attachments, and all the crural attachments were missing. Variations existed, but in some pups the stomach, spleen, and portions of the duodenum, pancreas, and liver were in the thoracic cavity.

Inheritance and Recommendation

The authors of the report stated that transmission of the defect could have been autosomal recessive, but due to limited data, other modes of gene action must be considered. This condition has been found to be inherited in other species.

If one accepts recessive inheritance, it should be dealt with as any other recessive.

REFERENCES

Feldman, D. B., and M. M. Bree. 1968. Congenital diaphragmatic hernia in neonatal dogs. JAVMA 153:942–44.

Fox, R. R., and D. D. Crary. 1973. Hereditary diaphragmatic hernia in the rabbit. J. Hered. 64:333–36.

Priester, W. A., A. G. Glass, and N. S. Waggoner. 1970. Congenital defects in domestic animals: General considerations. Am. J. Vet. Res. 31:1871–79.

GLOSSOPHARYNGEAL DEFECT (BIRD TONGUE)

A lethal glossopharyngeal hereditary defect has been reported in the dog. Unfortunately, the breed of dog was not revealed. Affected pups were born alive and at first observation appeared normal. Pups did not show an interest in nursing, even when aid was given, and died from starvation. Pups had unusually narrow tongues, could not swallow, and lacked the swallowing reflex. A very slight edema or fullness in the head was also reported. Since the pups did not attempt to suckle, it was difficult to evaluate their ability to do so.

Pathophysiology

Upon gross and microscopic observation, no abnormalities were reported other than the shape of the tongue. This was most evident in the rostral (anterior) half where the papillated margins were folded medially on the dorsal surface of the tongue.

It was not determined if the defect was an inability to swallow or if the tongue shape interfered with the suckling mechanism.

Inheritance and Recommendation

Genetic analyses showed the defect to result from an autosomal recessive.

One would select against such a trait as for any recessive gene. Homozygous recessive animals could not be used for testing since the condition is lethal, so one would use the known heterozygote.

REFERENCE

Hutt, F. B., and A. de Lahunta. 1971. A lethal glossopharyngeal defect in the dog. J. Hered. 62:291–93.

HERNIA (UMBILICAL AND INGUINAL)

The more frequent occurrence of umbilical and inguinal hernias in some breeds than in others suggests that the abnormality itself or some structural weakness resulting in a predisposition for hernia is heritable. Umbilical hernias are found in most breeds. Hereditary umbilical hernia has been reported in certain families of the collie, cocker spaniel, and bull terrier. One report indicated an increased risk of umbilical hernia in the Airedale, basenji, Pekingese, pointer, and Weimaraner.

For inguinal hernia a high breed incidence has been found in the basset hound, basenji, cairn terrier, Pekingese, and West Highland white terrier.

Some reports indicate that umbilical and inguinal hernias are inherited independently, while others are suggestive of a relationship between the two. The basenji and the Pekingese are high-risk breeds for both types.

Hernia may be observed soon after birth, depending somewhat on the severity, but often disappears as the dog matures.

Pathophysiology

According to the literature, canine umbilical hernia seems to be due to a failure of the normal occlusion of the umbilical ring, so that as the intra-abdominal pressure increases with the growth of the pup, the omentum and the intestines are forced through the aperture of the ring, pushing ahead the peritoneum covered by skin, thus producing a hernial sac containing one or both of the structures, usually small in the dog.

Also, for inguinal hernia (which in some reports includes scrotal hernia) the direct cause has been reported possibly to be an inherited factor affecting fibrous tissue and union of abdominal aponeuroses in the formation of the inguinal ring and linea alba. Weakness and defective formation of these structures would result in the appearance of the abnormalities.

Inheritance

Hernias appear in both sexes, but recent reports give a higher incidence of hernia in the bitch.

In the collie, cocker spaniel, and bull terrier, umbilical hernia is reported to be inherited independently of other forms of hernia and also independently of sex and color. For these breeds umbilical hernia is claimed to be due to a recessive gene, but multiple genetic factors may be involved.

For other breeds the type of gene action, the number of genes involved, the degree of penetrance, and the relationship among types of hernia may be the same as for the breeds listed above or may vary for the different breeds. This could account for the high incidence of umbilical hernias in the bitch and might suggest some type of sex-linked or partial sex-limited factor.

Recommendation

For breeding, do not use those animals that show the defect when mature or dogs that produce pups with a hernia. If the trait is recessive, additional test mating would be useful in eliminating the trait.

REFERENCES

Angus, K., and G. B. Young. 1972. A note on the genetics of umbilical hernia. Vet. Rec. 90:245–47.

Butler, H. C. 1960. Repair of congenital diaphragmatic hernia and umbilical hernia in a dog. JAVMA 136:559–60.

Catcott, E.J. 1966. Inherited abdominal defects in basenjis. Mod. Vet. Pract. 47(7):24.

Fox, M. W. 1963. Inherited inguinal hernia and midline defects in the dog. JAVMA 143:602–4.

Hayes, H.M., Jr. 1974. Congenital umbilical and inguinal hernias in cattle, horses, swine, dogs, and cats: Risk by breed and sex among hospital patients. Am. J. Vet. Res. 35:839–42.

Huron, L. 1961. Case reports: Mesh implant for correction of congenital midline hernia. Can. Vet. J. 2:393–96.

North, A. F., Jr. 1959. A new surgical approach to inguinal hernias in the dog. Cornell Vet. 49:378–83.

Phillips, J. McI., and T. M. Felton. 1939. Hereditary umbilical hernia in dogs. J. Hered. 30:433–35.

Priester, W. A., A. G. Glass, and N. S. Waggoner. 1970. Congenital defects in domesticated animals: General considerations. Am. J. Vet. Res. 31:1871–79.

Wright, J. G., II. 1963. The surgery of the inguinal canal in animals. Vet. Rec. 75:1352–63.

Section B:

DEFECTS WITH A POSSIBLE GENETIC BASE

SUMMARY OF DEFECTS

The following defects or abnormalities may well have a genetic base as indicated by breed predisposition or frequency of the defect in certain breeds or families, but data are less conclusive than for the defects previously discussed.

Sensory Organs
　　Dermoid cyst of cornea
　　Superficial indolent ulcer of cornea

Skeletal Anomalies
　　Cartilaginous exostoses
　　Craniomandibular osteopathy
　　Epiphyseal dysplasia
　　Foramen magnum
　　Hemivertebra
　　Intertarsal and tarso-metatarsal subluxation
　　Intervertebral disc degeneration
　　Aseptic necrosis of femoral head (Legg-Calvé-Perthes disease)
　　Osteogenesis imperfecta
　　Otocephaly
　　Panosteitis (enostoses)
　　Spondylosis deformans
　　Vertebral osteochondrosis

Neuromuscular System
　　Cerebrospinal demyelination
　　Cerebellar hypoplasia
　　Hydrocephalus
　　Trembling
　　Lissencephaly

Digestive System
Gingival hyperplasia

Endocrine and Metabolic Systems
Diabetes mellitus
Goiter
Glycogen storage disease

Urogenital System
Cystinuria
Familial renal disease
Renal agenesis

Skin
Canine hereditary black hair follicular dysplasia
Blue dog syndrome
Ectodermal defect
Hypotrichosis (hairlessness)

Other Structures
Calcinosis circumscripta
Laryngeal, tracheal collapse

CHAPTER 12

Sensory Organs

DERMOID CYST (CORNEA AND SCLERA)

A dermoid cyst appears as a tumorlike growth on the cornea or scleral conjuctiva. It usually consists of a skinlike structure (fibrofatty tissue covered by skin), with some of the structures of skin such as fibrous tissue, hair follicles, sebaceous glands, sweat glands, and fat, with one or more hairs projecting outward.

Dermoid cysts are more common in certain breeds, such as the German shepherd, Saint Bernard, Newfoundland, basset, dachshund, Welsh corgi, bulldog, cocker spaniel, and Weimaraner.

The condition results in a great deal of irritation, with resulting conjunctivitis and pannus (vascular proliferation) formation and occasionally interstitial keratitis.

Inheritance and Recommendation

If inherited, no mode of inheritance has been suggested. Since this condition is more frequent in certain breeds, indications are of at least a breed predisposed for it.

Without more information concerning the defect, recommendations cannot be made to decrease its frequency.

REFERENCES

Gelatt, K. N. 1971. Bilateral corneal dermoids and distichiasis in dogs. Vet. Med. Small Anim. Clin. 66:658–59.
Magrane, W. C. 1974. Canine ophthalmology, 2nd ed. Philadelphia: Lea & Febiger.

Lawson, D. D. 1975. Corneal dermoids in animals. Vet. Rec. 97:449–50.
Startup, F. G. 1969. Diseases of the Canine Eye. Baltimore: Williams & Wilkins.

SUPERFICIAL INDOLENT ULCER OF THE CORNEA

Superficial indolent ulcer is a corneal disease or defect peculiar to the boxer. The ulcer heals at one border but moves across the eye leaving scar tissue. The ulcer may persist for weeks or months and may be associated with endocrine or senile phenomena. The condition affects both sexes, is usually unilateral, and may be recurrent. Moderate pain is indicated by blepharospasm and watery or mucoid ocular discharge.

Pathophysiology

The superficial corneal ulcer is eccentric, benign, and indolent. There are no signs of iridocyclitis or hypopyon and no tendency toward perforation. The ulcer is shallow and round or oval, usually 2–3 mm from the corneoscleral limbus. The outer margin is more or less concentric with the limbus and there appears to be preference for the inferior (lower) part of the cornea.

Inheritance and Recommendation

Since more females have this disease than males, some type of sex or endocrine influence may be involved. No mode of inheritance is suggested, but it is probably an inherited trait since the condition is unique for the boxer.

Additional research must be conducted if one is to make positive recommendations concerning this trait.

REFERENCE

Roberts, S. R. 1965. Superficial indolent ulcer of the cornea in boxer dogs. J. Small Anim. Pract. 6:111–15.

CHAPTER 13

Bones and Joints

CARTILAGINOUS EXOSTOSES (ENCHONDROMATOSIS)

Cartilaginous exostoses is a condition in which bony growths project outward from the surface of the bone. Apparently the condition is rare. It has been reported most frequently in dogs of mixed breeding, but on one occasion in the Yorkshire terrier and in a malamute. Clinical signs include palpable masses located most frequently near the ends of long bones and ribs. Also in more advanced cases slight ataxia of the hindquarters and progressive posterior paresis occur.

The cause of exostoses is not established. Radiographically, multiple cartilaginous exostoses is a localized osteochondromatous outgrowth or expansion (an osseous mass) protruding from the bone. In dogs, exostoses have been found on the tibia, fibula, femur, ileum, radius, ulna, scapula, metatarsal bone, spinous processes of thoracic vertebrae, cervical vertebrae, spinous process of the atlas, and first phalanx. The lesions are covered by hyaline cartilage and are undergoing endochondral bone formation. They are of uneven size.

Inheritance and Recommendation

In the human, multiple cartilaginous exostoses is said to result from a dominant gene. It is also believed to be inherited in horses. In dogs, the mode of inheritance (if inherited) is not known. However, since progeny of an affected sire have shown the condition, the trait is probably inherited under some conditions.

Since the mode of genetic transmission is not known, it would be advisable not to use affected animals or close relatives of such animals in a breeding program.

REFERENCES

Banks, W. C., and C. H. Bridges. 1956. Multiple cartilaginous exostoses in a dog. JAVMA 129:131 35.

Carlson, W. D. 1967. Veterinary Radiology, 2nd ed. Philadelphia: Lea & Febiger.

Chester, D. K. 1971. Multiple cartilaginous exostoses in two generations of dogs. JAVMA 159:895-97.

Gee, B. R., and C. E. Doige. 1970. Multiple cartilaginous exostoses in a litter of dogs. JAVMA 156:53-59.

Owen, L. N., and D. E. Bostock. 1971. Multiple cartilaginous exostoses with development of a metastasizing osteosarcoma in a Shetland sheepdog. J. Small Anim. Pract. 12:507-12.

Owen, L. N., and S. W. Nielsen. 1968. Multiple cartilaginous exostoses (diaphyseal aclasis) in a Yorkshire terrier. J. Small Anim. Pract. 9:519-21.

Prata, R. G., S. G. Stoll, and F. A. Zaki. 1975. Spinal cord compression caused by osteocartilaginous exostoses of the spine in two dogs. JAVMA 166:371-75.

CRANIOMANDIBULAR OSTEOPATHY

Craniomandibular osteopathy, a disease characterized by bilateral irregular osseous proliferation of the mandible and tympanic bullae, is most often observed in the Scottish terrier and West Highland white terrier, but it has also been found in the Boston terrier, cairn terrier, and Labrador retriever. It is a disease of young dogs. Clinical signs are usually first observed between 4 and 7 months of age. Signs include an increase in the size of the lower jaw and difficulty in chewing or opening the mouth. Intermittent fever approaching 104° F also may be observed. The increase in size of the lower jaw is not regular. The condition is usually self limiting in that slowing and cessation of endochondral growth will occur.

Craniomandibular osteopathy affects the mandibles and the temporal and occipital bones. The histologic changes are characteristic, and they affect the cortical as well as the medullary trabeculae. They are produced in a haphazard combination of resorption and deposition. New deposits are coarse and poorly mineralized and show a random deposition. New deposits replace much of the original pattern of Haversian lamellae. Distinctive new and old bone in a histologic mosaic pattern are noticeable.

Inheritance and Recommendation

Due to the fact that this condition is more common in certain breeds, one would expect a genetic base. No mode of inheritance for this trait has been determined.

Avoid using affected animals or their close relatives for breeding.

REFERENCES

Jubb, K. V. F., and P. C. Kennedy. 1964. Pathology of domestic animals. New York: Academic Press, p. 40.

La Croix, J. A. 1970. Diagnosis of orthopedic problems peculiar to the growing dog. Vet. Med. Small Anim. Clin. 65:229-36.

Riser, W. H. 1966. What is your diagnosis? JAVMA 148:1543–47.
Riser, W. H., L. J. Parkers, and J. F. Shirer. 1967. Canine craniomandibular osteopathy. J. Am. Vet. Radiol. Soc. 8:23–31.
Littlewort, M. C. G. 1958. Tumorlike exostoses on the bone of head in puppies. Vet. Rec. 70:977–78.

EPIPHYSEAL DYSPLASIA

Epiphyseal dysplasia (stippled dysplasia, punctate epiphyseal dysplasia) has been reported in the beagle and miniature poodle. The condition is apparently rare but results in abnormal skeletal ossification. The entire skeleton may be involved, but the condition is more noticeable in the long bones. The condition may be noticed at birth, due to abnormal movements of the hind legs. Pups that survive have difficulty walking, have a swaying gait, fall easily, and appear to have a sagging at the joints and enlargement of the limbs. The difficulty of movement decreases with age. Many affected pups appear listless.

The condition is a form of chondrodystrophy characterized by the presence of numerous punctate areas of increased density in the epiphyses. Affected epiphyses are enlarged and dwarfism may result. In one report lesions were found bilaterally in the tarsal and carpal bones; in the femoral, humeral, metacarpal, and metatarsal epiphyses; and in the bodies of the sixth and seventh lumbar vertebrae. In a second report the condition appeared even more widespread.

Inheritance and Recommendation

If inherited, the mode or type of inheritance was not suggested.

The only recommendation one could make with such limited data would be to avoid breeding affected animals or their close relatives.

REFERENCES

Cotchin, E., and K. M. Dyce. 1956. A case of epiphyseal dysplasia in a dog. Vet. Rec. 68:427–28.
Hanlon, G. F. 1962. Normal and abnormal bone growth in the dog. J. Am. Vet. Radiol. Soc. 3:13–16.
Lodge, D. 1966. Two cases of epiphyseal dysplasia. Vet. Rec. 79:136–38.
Rasmussen, P. G. 1971. Multiple epiphyseal dysplasia in a litter of beagle puppies. J. Small Anim. Pract. 12:91–96.
_____. 1972. Multiple epiphyseal dysplasia in beagle puppies. Acta Radiol. Suppl. 319, pp. 251–54.

FORAMEN MAGNUM

A malformation of the occipital bone with enlargement of the foramen magnum has been observed in Chihuahuas, cocker spaniels, and Skye terriers. Some dogs have no symptoms at all, while others appear to have pain over the occipitocervical region. Frequent scratching of the ear is common. The tongue may protrude from the mouth, with loss of pain sensation in the tongue. Pawing at the face is also noted. In pups, the sign of dorsal spinal cord involvement may be observed. Unsteadiness of forelegs is noted. Sudden temporary changes in the dog's temperament may occur. Signs may be first observed in the young pup or may not appear until the dog is fully mature.

Pathophysiology

With the defect, the foramen extends dorsally to within a few millimeters of the external occipital crest, resulting in the absence of a nuchal tubercle. This extension of the foramen magnum past its usual limits results in exposure of the cerebellum and brain stem. In the young pup with posterior displacement of the neural structures, there is an enlargement of the ventricles with hydrocephalus and neurologic signs. Hydrocephalus is not observed in older dogs with neurologic signs. In some cases the hind brain extends beyond the occipital bone and the brain stem lies within the atlas and axis (first two cervical vertebrae).

Inheritance and Recommendation

No mode of inheritance was suggested, only that there were indications of an inherited condition.

Since the mode of inheritance is not defined, a detailed breeding program cannot be suggested. Avoid the use of an affected dog or its close relatives in a breeding program.

REFERENCE

Bardens, J. W. 1965. Congenital malformation of the foramen magnum in dogs. Southwest. Vet. 18:295-98.

HEMIVERTEBRA (BUTTERFLY VERTEBRA)

Hemivertebra refers to a condition usually observed in small and brachycephalic breeds (screw-tailed breeds such as English bulldogs, French bulldogs, and Boston terriers, and also pugs and Pomeranians) in which one observes wedge-shaped vertebra. Often clinical signs are not observed, but clinically one may observe a progressive hind leg weakness (due to spinal cord pressure, which may affect one leg more than the other), spinal pain, abnormalities of the nervous system (urinary and fecal inconsistencies), and evidence of muscle atrophy, etc. Signs of the presence of kyphosis or scoliosis (curved spine) are usually observed by the time the dog reaches 1 year of age.

The defect results from an abnormal development of individual vertebrae due to failure of fusion of the centers of ossification of the right and left halves of the vertebral bodies. This asymmetric development of the individual vertebrae has been said to be due to the persistence of a midline septum arising from a perichondral sheath remnant around the notochord. The abnormalities may appear in a number of forms, affecting the structure and/or function of the vertebra in a number of ways. The condition may exist anywere in the spine, but the vertebrae most commonly affected were in the region T7–9. They may appear to be spread and resemble a butterfly.

Inheritance and Recommendation

The increased frequency of the condition in families of dogs suggests that it might be inherited.

Do not include an affected dog in breeding programs.

REFERENCES

Done, S. H., R. A. Drew, G. M. Robins, and J. G. Lane. 1975. Hemivertebra in the dog: Clinical and pathological observations. Vet. Rec. 96:313–17.

Drew, R. A. 1974. Possible association between abnormal vertebral development and neonatal mortality in bulldogs. Vet. Rec. 94:480–81.

Grenn, H. H., and D. E. Lindo. 1969. Hemivertebrae with severe kypho-scoliosis and accompanying deformities in a dog. Can. Vet. J. 10:214–16.

Hoerlein, B. F. 1971. Canine neurology: Diagnosis and treatment, 2nd ed. Philadelphia: W. B. Saunders.

Morgan, J. P. 1968. Congenital anomalies of the vertebral column of the dog. A study of the incidence and significance based on a radiographic and morphologic study. J. Am. Vet. Radiol. Soc. 9:21–29.

Olsson, S. D. 1965. Canine surgery. First Archibald Edition. American Veterinary Publications. Wheaton and Santa Barbara, U.S.A. 868.

Putman, R. W., and J. Archibald. 1968. Canine medicine. First Catcott Edition. American Veterinary Publications. Wheaton and Santa Barbara, U.S.A. 498, 686.

INTERTARSAL AND TARSOMETATARSAL SUBLUXATION

These subluxations occur in many breeds. However, it would appear that the Shetland sheepdog (England) is predisposed to intertarsal subluxation. The condition is also reported to be common in the collie. Intertarsal subluxation primarily involves the intertarsal joint (between first and second rows of tarsal bones) but sometimes the area between the fibular and tibial bones. Tarsometatarsal subluxation occurs less frequently. The traumatic event usually imitates its condition.

Dogs with intertarsal subluxation usually show moderate to severe lameness and abnormal angulation (dorsiflexion) of the hock joint; an unstable joint may be observed. The chronically affected animal shows a thickening of the joint. The condition may be bilateral. The development of the condition in both legs does not occur at the same time.

For the sheltie a very specific age incidence (6–9 years) was observed. Age varied more in other breeds.

The vast majority of cases involve the proximal intertarsal joint (39 cases of 54). Two occurred at the distal intertarsal joint and 3 showed separation between the tibial and fibular tarsal bones (proximal intratarsal joint). It was reported that at least in the case of the Shetland sheepdog, the dogs had suffered a gradual degeneration of the plantar ligament.

Tarsometatarsal subluxation occurred only when the strong tarsometatarsal joint capsule, which is reinforced by the attachment of the plantar ligament, is torn. This usually results from some form of trauma.

Inheritance and Recommendation

The data given suggest that the Shetland sheepdog is prone to proximal intertarsal subluxation. No mode of gene action is suggested, but the higher incidence in the sheltie and collie does suggest a genetic pattern. Environment does interact, since the majority of cases were in the larger, heavier dogs.

Avoid including individuals with this condition in breeding programs. Screen closely related animals.

REFERENCES

Campbell, J. R., D. Bennett, and R. Lee. 1976. Intertarsal and tarso-metatarsal subluxation in the dog. J. Small Anim. Pract. 17:427–42.
Clayton-Jones, D. G. 1974. Hindleg lameness in the dog. In Veterinary Annual, 14th ed. Edited by C. S. G. Grunsell and F. W. G. Hill. P. 167. Bristol: John Wright and Sons.
Lawson, D. D. 1961. Intertarsal subluxation in the dog. J. Small Anim. Pract. 1:179–81.

INTERVERTEBRAL DISC DEGENERATION

Certain breeds of dogs appear to have a predisposition for intervetebral (IV) disc protrusion. The incidence is highest in the chondrodystrophoid breeds, but the condition also occurs in others. In various studies the condition was found in 84 breeds (varieties). This condition is very common in the dachshund, Pekingese, French bulldog, American cocker, beagle, Welsh corgi, Lhasa Apso, miniature poodle, and Shih Tzu.

Symptoms vary a great deal. Intermittent symptoms or remission may occur. The stages of symptoms have been classified as pain, paresis, incoordination, paralysis (spastic or flaccid), and progressive ascending paralysis consequent to extensive rupture of the disc and generalized hemorrhage in the cord.

Two types of disc protrusion apparently exist: the first type, that of the chondrodystrophoid breeds, the type in which heredity may be important; and the second type, a senile form. In the first type, disc protrusion is preceded by a chondroid metamorphosis of the nucleus pulposus (center of the IV disc), rather uniformly distributed in the vertebral column. At approximately 1 year of age, 75%-100% of the nuclei have been transformed into a chondroid tissue of hyaline type, 30%-60% of them showing macroscopic signs of degeneration, mainly in the form of calcification. The nucleus pulposus begins to lose its mucoid nature during the first year, and by 4 years of age the nucleus has become cartilaginous and often calcified. The annulus fibrosus (periphery of the disc) also undergoes structural alteration. The lamellae loosen and disintegrate or become hyalinized. As the disc loses its original structure, its ability to function as a shock absorber decreases along with its ability to receive adequate nutrition. The degenerate disc's inability to withstand day-to-day activity allows increasing liability to injury such as annulus fibrosus and dorsal spinal ligament rupture, thus allowing the nucleus pulposus material to be extruded. This is most prominent in the chondrodystrophoid breeds in which the degenerative changes are advanced at an age when the dog is still active. The most likely location for disc protrusion by the nucleus pulposus is via the dorsal annulus and into the neural canal, since the annulus is weakened and is thinnest dorsally. Disc protrusions most commonly occur at or near the thoracolumbar junction.

In senile degeneration the nucleus pulposus gradually becomes fibrous as a result of collagenization, but usually this process is advanced to significant proportions at an older age (7 or more years). The senile type takes place independently of breed.

Inheritance and Recommendation

No genetic pattern has been proved. The fact that certain breeds have a high incidence is quite suggestive of an inheritable trait, either directly or indirectly due to breed conformation.

Careful selection against affected animals is all that can be suggested when the type of gene action is not known.

REFERENCES

Braund, K. G., P. Ghosh, T. K. F. Taylor, and L. H. Larsen. 1975. Morphological studies of the canine intervertebral disc. The assignment of the beagle to the achondroplastic classification. Res. Vet. Sci. 19:167-72.

Ghosh, P., T. K. F. Taylor, J. M. Yarrell, K. G. Braund, and L. H. Larsen. 1975. Genetic factors in the maturation of the canine intervertebral disc. Res. Vet. Sci. 19:304-11.

Hansen, H. J. 1959. Comparative views on the pathology of disc degeneration in animals. Lab. Invest. 8:1242-65.

_____. 1964. The body constitution of dogs and its importance for the occurrence of disease. Nord. Vet. Med. 16:977-87.

Hoerlein, B. F. 1971. Canine neurology: Diagnosis and treatment, 2nd ed. Philadelphia, London, Toronto: W. B. Saunders.

Priester, W. A. 1976. Canine intervertebral disc disease: Occurrence by age, breed, and sex among 8,117 cases. Theriogenology 6:293–303.

Russell, S. W., and R. C. Griffiths. 1968. Recurrence of cervical disc syndrome in surgically and conservatively treated dogs. JAVMA 153:1412.

Vaughan, L. C. 1958. Studies on intervertebral disc protrusion in the dog. Br. Vet. J. 114:105–12.

ASCEPTIC NECROSIS OF FEMORAL HEAD (LEGG-CALVÉ-PERTHES DISEASE)

Legg-Calvé-Perthes disease refers to a juvenile aseptic (ischemic) necrosis of the femoral head. It is a disease of the small breeds, especially the wirehaired terriers, Manchester terriers, miniature and toy poodles, miniature schanuzers, pugs, and Pekingese. This condition has been reported in breeds as large as the cocker and Shetland sheepdog. Clinical signs are usually first observed in pups between 3 and 11 months of age. Clinical signs include chronic hind leg lameness of sudden onset, which becomes somewhat less as the dog gets older. Evidence of pain occurs when manipulating the joint, weight is shifted to the front legs, leg motion is reduced, and some muscle atrophy may occur. Either leg may be affected and in some cases both legs are involved.

The lesion begins as an increase in trabecular (spongy) bone in the head of the femur, followed by aseptic necrosis. The necrosis results from a lack of blood supply (ischemia). Initially the bones show increased density due to the ischemia, but later revascularization is accompanied by decalcification of the dead bone. At this stage the bone is soft and easily broken. Later the bone recalcifies but usually does not obtain its former state. Growth of the epiphyseal cartilage may be impaired, causing the femoral neck to be shorter and thicker as a result of abnormal productive bone. This results in poor feet and possible osteoarthritis.

Inheritance and Recommendation

The condition affects both sexes. Certain families show a high incidence of the disease. A specific genetic factor has not been proved.

The use of such animals for breeding is not suggested.

REFERENCES

La Croix, J. A. 1970. Diagnosis of orthopedic problems peculiar to the growing dog. Vet. Med. Small Anim. Clin. 65:229–36.

Lee, R., and P. D. Fry. 1969. Some observations on the occurrence of Legg-Calvé-Perthes disease (coxaplana) in the dog, and an evaluation of excision arthroplasty as a method of treatment. J. Small Anim. Pract. 10:309–17.

Ljunggren, G. 1967. Legg-Perthes disease in the dog. Acta Orthop. Scand. Suppl. 94.

Paatsama, S., P. Rissanen, and P. Robbanen. 1967. Biochemical changes in Legg-Perthes disease. J. Small Anim. Pract. 8:215–20.

Phillips, T. N., and D. Maksic. 1963. Idiopathic osteonecrosis of the femoral head. Mod. Vet. Pract. 44(2):56–57.

Riser, W. H. 1963. Necrosis of the femoral head. JAVMA 142:1021–24.
Smith, K. W. 1971. Legg-Perthes disease. Vet. Clin. of North Am. 1(3):479–87.

OSTEOGENESIS IMPERFECTA
(SECONDARY HYPERPARATHYROIDISM)

Osteogenesis imperfecta is a condition representing a deficient or delayed developmental formation of bone, believed to result from a deficiency of osteoblasts. It has been found in standard poodles, Norwegian elkhounds, and Bedlington terriers. Clinical manifestations are skeletal abnormalities, usually of the spinal column and posterior extremities. Numerous fractures occur. The fractures result from minor injury or trauma but heal rapidly. Deformities are characterized by a flattening of the front paws and metatarsal bones, creating a snowshoe appearance, an outward bowing of the elbow, and a severe knock-kneed appearance. Also there is a striking flaccidity of the ligaments and joints. Abnormalities are apparent at 6–8 weeks of age, and abnormal characteristics usually improve at puberty.

Involved bones showed very thin cortices, thin and sparse cancellous bone (especially in the area of the metaphyses), and fractures occurring through almost every metaphysis. The bones of affected dogs appear to lag behind normal individuals in development by 1–2 months (an inhibition or delay of osteogenesis). Two important deviations from normal were observed: a definite narrowing of the epiphyseal plate, apparently due to a diminution in the numbers of both the proliferating and degenerating cartilage cells; and second, a decrease in the activity and the number of osteoblasts and sparseness and thinness of the trabeculae.

Inheritance and Recommendation

The family history of the pups considered in these studies suggests a genetic background to the condition. No mode of inheritance is suggested.

Recommendations other than careful selection of breeding animals cannot be given on such limited data.

REFERENCES

Calkins, E., D. Kalm, and W. C. Diner. 1956. Idiopathic familial osteoporosis in dogs: "Osteogenesis imperfecta." Ann. N.Y. Acad. Sci. 64(3):410–23.
Lettow, E., and K. Dammrich. 1960. Beitrog zur klink und Pathologie der osteogenesis imperfecta bei junghunden. Zentralbl. Veterinaermed. 7:962–63.

OTOCEPHALY

The medical dictionary describes otocephalus as a monster fetus lacking the lower jaw and having ears united below the face. This condition is not common in the dog, but variations (aprosopic—part of face missing) of the defect have been observed for many years. Pups born with this as a severe defect would normally be short lived.

Authors are not all in agreement as to what constitutes an "otocephalic syndrome," and the degree thereof. Low-grade otocephalics would not be lethal.

Pathophysiology

If one accepts the strict medical definition as absolute, then the defect would be a pup without a lower jaw and with ears united below the face, or if one accepts grades or degrees of otocephaly, the following has been given: A high grade of otocephaly is where aprosopus is found. Several structures cephalad (anterior) to the medulla are deficient. The eye, cerebral cortex, maxillae, and mandibles are absent. Intermediate forms are found with shortened lower jaw, cyclopia, and ears anastamosed in the midventral line. Low-grade otocephaly would be agnathia (short lower jaw) with secondary hydrocephaly.

Inheritance and Recommendation

Low-grade otocephaly as described by some authors was said to be inherited. Distinction made between low- and high-grade otocephaly would suggest multigenetic factors.

Eliminate affected and closely related animals from breeding stock.

REFERENCES

Fox, M. W. 1963. Low-grade otocephaly in a dog. JAVMA 143:289–90.
_____. 1963. Developmental abnormalities of the canine skull. Can. J. Comp. Med. 27:219–22.
_____. 1964. Anatomy of the canine skull in low-grade otocephaly. Can. J. Comp. Med. 28:105–7.
_____. 1964. The otocephalic syndrome in the dog. Cornell Vet. 54:250–59.
Kalter, H. 1968. Teratology of the central nervous system. Chicago and London: Univ. of Chicago Press.

PANOSTEITIS (ENOSTOSIS)

Panosteitis is a condition that for the most part affects the long bones. This condition usually becomes noticeable between the ages of 5 and 12 months. Reportedly it is most common in the German shepherd.

Clinical signs include lameness, usually lasting for a few days or a week. The expressed pain may shift after a 1–3-week duration to other locations (limbs). The condition is benign and disappears spontaneously, usually before 18 months of age but in some cases lasts much longer.

The bone most often affected is the ulna, followed by the humerus, radius, and tibia. Histopathologic findings have shown excessive formation of bones of various degrees of maturity throughout the long bone and excessive osteoblastic activity with formation of bone by fibrous metaplasia.

Enostosis was revealed, subperiosteal new bone formation, and in some bones cortical changes of an osteolytic nature. Osteoblastic and osteoclastic activities were observed surrounding the remodeled Haversian system. On occasion the cavernous cortical remodeling blended into the endosteal and periosteal reactions.

Three zones of reaction were recognized by cellular arrangement. The cortical cells were arranged in longitudinal fashion, with the periosteal reaction perpendicular to it. The endosteal reaction was arranged in haphazard fashion and was easily recognized and differentiated from cortical bones.

Inheritance and Recommendation

The condition is reported to be most common in the male. In one study the incidence of the condition in a colony of dogs that were progeny of affected dogs was 100%. As stated, this does not prove the existence of a genetic factor but does at least suggest an increased inherent susceptibility.

With an uncertain genetic pattern, one cannot give detailed recommendations. Carefully screen breeding animals and avoid including affected animals where possible.

REFERENCES

Barrett, R. B., W. D. Schall, and R. E. Lewis. 1968. Clinical and radiographic features of canine eosinophilic panosteitis. JAAHA 4:94–104.

Bohning, B. H., P. F. Sutter, B. Hohn, and J. L. Marshall. 1970. Clinical and radiological survey of canine panosteitis. JAVMA 156:870–83.

Burt, J. K., and G. P. Wilson, III. 1972. A study of eosinophilic panosteitis (enostosis) in the German shepherd dog. Acta Radiol. Suppl. 319, pp. 7–13.

Cotter, S. M., R. C. Griffiths, and I. Lear. 1968. Enostosis of young dogs. JAVMA 153:401–10.

Evers, W. H. 1969. Enostosis in a dog. JAVMA 154:799–803.

Kasstrom, H., Sten-Erik Olsson, and P. F. Sutter. 1972. Panosteitis in the dog. Acta Radiol. Suppl. 319, pp. 15–23.

Zeskor, B. 1962. A contribution to eosinophylic panosteitis in German shepherd dogs. Veterinarski Arkiv, Zagreb, Knjuga, XXXII, Svezak 5-6, pp. 146–49. Yrednistvo Primilo Rukopis 10, II, 1962.

SPONDYLITIS DEFORMANS

Spondylitis deformans refers to a condition in the intervertebral space in which there is an inflammation of the vertebral joints and a degeneration mainly in the ventral part of the discs, resulting in the outgrowth of bonelike spurs on the borders of the vertebral bodies. These spurs may fuse, causing ankylosis. The term spondylitis deformans is used interchangeably with spinal osteoarthritis. Spinal osteoarthritis is usually observed in older dogs. Clinical signs may be stiffness, soreness, and reduced movements of the back legs.

The condition is observed in most breeds but not in the boxer, cocker, Airedale, German shepherd, or French bulldog. The condition in the dachshund is variably reported as both high and low incidence by different workers.

Pathophysiology

Any vertebrae may be affected, but the ones most commonly affected are the last two or three thoracic and the lumbar vertebrae. The spur develops on one of the articular margins of the vertebral body, causing progressive fusing and fixation of the joint.

Inheritance and Recommendation

If the condition is inherited, no type of gene action is suggested. The more frequent occurrence of the defect in certain different conformations suggests a possible genetic base.

A breeding program should consider the possibility of a genetic factor, but without a more clear-cut genetic pattern specific recommendations cannot be made.

REFERENCES

Glenney, W. C. 1956. Canine and feline spinal osteoarthritis (spondylitis deformans). JAVMA 129:61–66.
Hansen, H. J. 1959. Comparative views on the pathology of disc degeneration in animals. Lab. Invest. 8:1242–65.
Morgan, J. P., G. Ljunggren, and R. Read. 1967. Spondylosis deformans (vertebral osteophytosis) in the dog. J. Small Anim. Pract. 8:57–66.

VERTEBRAL OSTEOCHONDROSIS

This condition has been reported in the foxhound. It is characterized by an arching of the back (thoracolumbar spine), which becomes prominent owing to the loss of paraspinal muscle, a stilted hind leg movement with the pelvis elevated above the shoulders, and general unthriftiness. Lesions are usually first observed at approximately 7–10 months of age.

Pathophysiology

The defect appears to be associated with the degeneration of the intervertebral disc, and the following clinical signs are observed: the erosion of the cancellous bone of the varying vertebral bodies, with a resultant narrowing of the intervertebral space, exostoses (outgrowth) on the ventral surface of the vertebrae, and exostoses and ankylosis (fusion of vertebrae affecting intervertebral movement).

Dislocation of the disc material or cartilage end-plate of the vertebral body may exist; a part of the nucleus pulposus is propelled through the end-plate into the underlying bone of the vertebral centrum, in a cranial or caudal direction. This leads to the formation of pits in the body of the vertebra. The condition then progresses to exostoses, which may ankylose ventral to the vertebral body.

Inheritance and Recommendation

A mode of inheritance is not reported, but known affected pups were all from one sire. A genetic condition is indicated.

Cull defective animals. Do not use close relatives in the breeding program.

REFERENCES

Ghosh, P., T. K. F. Taylor, J. M. Yarrell, K. G. Braund, and L. H. Larsen. 1975. Genetic factors in the maturation of the canine intervertebral disc. Res. Vet. Sci. 19:304–11.

Hansen, H. J. 1959. Comparative views on the pathology of disc degeneration in animals. Lab. Invest. 8:1242–65.

_____. 1963. An unusual spinal condition in foxhounds. Vet. Rec. 75:644.

Hime, J. M., and J. C. Drake. 1965. Osteochrondroses of the spine in the foxhound. Vet. Rec. 77:445–49.

CHAPTER 14

Neuromuscular System

CEREBROSPINAL DEMYELINATION

Cerebrospinal demyelination, a primary demyelinating disease, has been reported in the miniature poodle between 9 weeks and 5 months of age.

Pups initially have difficulty standing on the hind limbs a spastic type of paraplegia develops, which later involves the forelimbs, resulting in ataxic and abnormal posture and usually death.

Abnormalities appear confined to the central nervous system. The principal pathologic abnormalities were large areas of demyelination in the tegmentum and upper cervical cord, with smaller foci bilaterally distributed in the brain stem. Long tracts appeared to be particularly affected. The process is essentially a destruction of myelin rather than a hypomyelinogenesis.

Inheritance and Recommendation

The condition in one report occurred in full sibs. No genetic conclusions or recommendation could be made without a great deal more information.

REFERENCES

Douglas, S. W., and A. C. Palmer. 1961. Idiopathic demyelination of brain-stem and spinal cord in a miniature poodle puppy. J. Pathol. Bactiol. 82:67–71.

McGrath, J. T. 1960. Neurologic examination of the dog with clinicopathologic observations, 2nd ed. Philadelphia: Lea & Febiger.

Steinberg, S. A. 1963. Clinicopathologic conference. J. Am. Vet. Med. Assoc. 143:404–10.

CEREBELLAR HYPOPLASIA

An unusual cerebellar ataxia has been reported in a family of Airedales.

The condition was first observed when the pups approached 12 weeks of age. The condition was progressive. When walking, the legs flopped and jerked erratically, and on occasion the animal would fall. During walking the forelegs would be lifted high and then suddenly thrust forward to an excessive distance. Animals would experience difficulty in standing, but could sit; however, even while sitting they exhibited a marked swaying of the head and trunk.

Pathophysiology

The main microscopic lesion reported was an absence and degeneration of the Purkinje cells. In all parts of the cortex less than 5% of the original number remained. Probably both hypoplasia and degeneration occurred. Neuroblasts were numerous in the molecular layer.

Limited gliosis was confined to the Purkinje and molecular strata. Demyelination was absent.

Inheritance and Recommendation

The relationship between affected dogs suggests a hereditary condition, but on such limited observations one could not state a mode of inheritance or make recommendations other than to avoid using animals closely related to affected ones in a breeding program.

REFERENCE

Cordy, D. R., and H. A. Snelbaker. 1952. Cerebellar hypoplasia and degeneration in a family of Airedale dogs. J. Neuropathol. Exp. Neurol. 11:324–28.

HYDROCEPHALUS

Hydrocephalus is a defect or condition that is characterized by an excessive accumulation of cerebral fluid. Most cases of hydrocephalus occur in the miniature breeds of dogs with dome-shaped heads. Examples would be the Chihuahua, Manchester terrier, and the Pekingese. Brachycephalic breeds are also subject to hydrocephalus. Clinical signs are multiple and varied. Hydrocephalic signs may be apparent in the very young pup. The head is enlarged and the open fontanelles can be detected on palpation. The skull enlarges to accommodate the increased volume of fluid. Affected pups may show depressed neurologic activity, dullness, inactivity, stupidity, or locomotor weakness, or they may whine a great deal. Brain reflexes and spinal reflexes are abnormal. Various visual deficits are observed.

Pathophysiology

Any condition that contributes to excessive accumulation of fluid such as overproduction, deficiency of absorption, or altered flow of cerebrospinal fluid will result in hydrocephalus. This condition may be secondarily caused in the cranium as a result of abnormal accumulation of cerebrospinal fluid in the lateral ventricles of the cerebral hemispheres. The cerebrospinal fluid is unable to circulate through openings that normally occur in the roof of the fourth ventricle of the medulla oblongata. This stoppage may result from an accumulation of proteinaceous material in the foraminas through which the fluid should flow. The closure of the dermal bones that form the calvarium is delayed, and the skull becomes enlarged.

Inheritance and Recommendation

In some cases of hydrocephalus, genetics may be involved. Hydrocephalus may be secondary in certain conformations in breeds selected for that characteristic, e.g., brachycephalic breeds. This implies a genetic relationship, even when effects are secondary. Also, in one colony of beagles the defect, along with other abnormalities, was considered dependent largely upon genetic factors. A low degree of hydrocephaly has been reported in cockers.

In breeds where conformation does not encourage the defect, do not include such animals and close relatives in a breeding program.

REFERENCES

Fuller, J. L. 1956. The inheritance of structural defects in dogs. Michigan State Univ. Vet. 16:103–8, 125.

Gage, E. D., and B. F. Hoerlein. 1968. Surgical treatment of canine hydrocephalus by ventriculoatrial shunting. JAVMA 153:1418–31.

Green, E. L. 1957. Mutant stock of cats and dogs offered for research. J. Hered. 48:56–57.

Hoerlein, B. F. 1971. Canine Neurology, 2nd ed. Philadelphia: W. B. Saunders.

Innes, J. R. M., and L. Z. Saunders. 1962. Comparative Neuropathology. New York: Academic Press.

Kalter, H. 1968. Teratology of the Central Nervous System. Chicago and London: Univ. of Chicago Press.

Scott, J. P., and Fuller, J. L. 1965. Genetics and the social behavior of the dog. Chicago and London: Univ. of Chicago Press.

Stockard, C. R. 1941. The genetic and endocrinic basis for differences in form and behavior as elucidated by studies of contrasted pure-line dog breeds and hybrids. American Anatomical Memoirs. Philadelphia: Wistar Institute of Anatomy and Biology.

TREMBLING

A condition referred to as trembling was reported in one Airedale terrier. Trembling of the hind limb and tail was of long duration but did not occur when the dog slept. Since this defect was reported for only one dog, one could not even suggest this to be an inherited trait. However, the dog with the trembling condition was inbred and traced several times to one ancestor.

REFERENCE

Kollarits, J. 1924. Permanent trembling in some dog breeds as hereditary degeneration. Schweiz. Med. Wochenschr. 54:431–32.

LISSENCEPHALY

Lissencephaly, a condition characterized by the absence of or a limited number of cerebracortical convolutions, has been reported in two Lhasa Apso dogs.

Seizures of the grand mal type lasting 2–3 minutes were observed. Postictal events were characterized by behavioral alterations, hunger, confusion, and intermittent blindness. The frequency of seizure was initially 1–2 per week, but at a later age seizures increased to several times a day. The dogs' behavior toward people was reported to be one of apprehension and seclusion. Occasionally the dogs were depressed and confused but at other times were active. At times they were aggressive and did not appear to recognize their owner and attacked the owner. When running, the dogs on occasion ran into stationary objects. They occasionally assumed an unusual posture, with hind limbs abducted when lying down. Also, in one of the dogs, postural reactions including wheelbarrowing, optic and taclite pacing, hopping, extensor postural thrust, and hemiwalking were slow in all limbs.

Pathophysiology

The most remarkable finding was an almost complete lack of convolutions on the cerebrum.

Inheritance and Recommendation

The authors did not suggest any genetic pattern. The animals were not closely related, but, since they were of the same breed, a genetic basis for the disorder should have been considered. The occurrence of this condition in some species lends support for a genetic basis.

Genetic recommendation cannot be made based on information from only two individuals. Avoid close relatives of such an animal in a breeding program if possible.

REFERENCE

Green, C. E., M. Vandevelde, and K. Braund. 1976. Lissencephaly in two Lhasa Apso dogs. JAVMA 169(4):405–10.

CHAPTER 15

Digestive System

GINGIVAL HYPERTROPHY

Gingival hypertrophy is reported in four related male boxers. Raised areas may be noted at various locations along the gum line. Both jaws may be affected.

Lesions are characterized by a central area of bone and by nests and cords of cells suggestive of odontogenic epithelium.

Inheritance and Recommendation

Conclusions cannot be drawn on such a limited number of animals. A genetic involvement could be indicated since animals involved were closely related.

If this condition occurs, screen affected and related animals from breeding programs.

REFERENCES
Burstone, M. S., E. Bond, and R. Litt. 1952. Familial gingival hypertrophy in the dog (boxer breed). Arch. Pathol. 54:208–12.

CHAPTER 16

Endocrine and Metabolic Systems

DIABETES MELLITUS

In the dog, the influence of genetics on diabetes is not well documented. Since heredity appears to play an important role in the human, it seems reasonable to assume a genetic relationship may be involved in the dog. Diabetes occurs in most breeds, but in one study a high incidence was found in the dachshund that may well indicate a familial tendency. Noticeable signs include loss of weight, increased thirst, and excessive urination. In the dog, diabetes is reported more often in the female. Most cases occur in older dogs (5–12 years), with the peak age being 8–9 years of age.

Pathophysiology

The basic cause is a deficiency of insulin at the cellular level. The exact mechanism of insulin action is unknown, but it is believed that the lack of insulin renders the glucose incapable of moving across the membrane of certain cells. The result is hyperglycemia or increased blood sugar. This quickly leads to glycosuria or sugar in the urine accompanied by excessive urination and increased thirst. Since the animal is unable to use carbohydrates as an energy source, the body attempts to supply needed energy by the breakdown of protein, which results in nitrogen loss and body weight loss and the breakdown of fat. Fat breakdown increases the supply of ketone bodies, which are acid, and since the ketone bodies are now in excess they must be buffered. This taxes the acid-base balance system, which leads to acidosis and dehydration and, together with polyuria, results in a loss of electrolytes. If not treated, severe cases result in coma and death.

Inheritance and Recommendation

As mentioned above in the human, heredity plays an important role in the occurrence of diabetes mellitus. In the dog the influence of genetics is not well documented. It seems reasonable to assume a genetic relationship may be involved.

Because of the uncertainty of the role of genetics in dog diabetes, one cannot make an absolute recommendation. Avoid the use of affected and close relatives of affected animals in breeding programs.

REFERENCES

Joshua, J. O. 1963. Some clinical aspects of diabetes mellitus in the dog and cat. J. Small Anim. Pract. 4:275–80.
Keen, H. 1960. Spontaneous diabetes in man and animals. Vet. Rec. 72:555–58.
Wilkinson, J. S. 1960. Spontaneous diabetes mellitus. Vet. Rec. 72:548–55.

GOITER

Goiter was found in a family of fox terriers. Clinical signs and physiopathology were as expected. Since the goiter was found in 6 of 23 offspring from one dam, an indication of a genetic background to the condition resulted.

REFERENCE

Brouwers, J. 1950. Goitre et heredite chez le chien. Ann. Med. Vet. 94:173–74.

GLYCOGEN STORAGE DISEASE

Glycogen storage disease (initiated by stress) is a rare condition similar to the von Gierke syndrome in humans.

The condition is confined to pups of the toy breed and usually appears between 6 and 12 weeks of age.

One observes depression and muscular tremor, signs of vertigo and incoordination, retraction of the eye, a sunken appearance of the upper eyelid, coma, a decrease in temperature, and a decrease in blood glucose.

Histopathologic studies reveal glycogen infiltration of the visceral organs. The hepatic cells are enlarged and the sinusoids compressed while the epithelia of the renal tubules are swollen with a decrease in lumina. Some pups had excessive glycogen deposits in the myocardium. There may be three forms of glycogen storage disease. The first, which includes most cases, is a generalized disease; second, a von Gierke-like syndrome resulting from a glucose 6-phosphatase (enzyme) deficiency; and third, Cori's disease (limited dextrinosis), a deficiency of amylo-1, 6-phosphatase.

Inheritance and Recommendation

Direct evidence for an inherited condition is not given; however, many of the pups showing the condition were reported to be related.

Without direct evidence of a genetic relationship, specific recommendations cannot be made.

REFERENCES

Bardens, J. W. 1966. Glycogen storage disease in puppies. Vet. Med. Small Anim. Clin. 61:1174-76.

Bardens, J. W., G. Bardens, and B. Bardens. 1961. A von Gierke-like syndrome. Allied Vet. 32:4-7.

Mostafa, I. E. 1970. A case of glycogenic cardiomegaly in a dog. Acta Vet. Scand. 11:197-208.

CHAPTER 17

Urogenital System

CYSTINURIA

Cystinuria is a condition in which (1) cystine is excreted in the urine due to an anomoly of renal tubular transport of cystine and possibly other amino acids, and (2) urinary calculi may result because of the insolubility of cystine in the urine.

Canine cystinuria accounts for approximately 10% of the urinary calculi in dogs. The condition appears to be most common in the dachshund, but occurs in many breeds. The first attack of urethral obstruction usually occurs between 1½ and 3 years of age.

Pathophysiology

Literature indicates that there are two populations of cystinuric dogs—one with a lysine and cystine defect and one with a cystine defect only. *In vitro* studies show the defect to be a renal tubule reabsorption defect.

Inheritance and Recommendation

The mode of genetic transmission of the disease is presently unclear. Since the condition does occur more often in certain breeds than others and since closely related dogs have been reported to have the defect, a genetically controlled condition is probable. Because the condition has been reported in males only, it may be a sex-linked trait.

It is difficult to recommend a breeding program for traits suggested as heritable in some unknown way. However, general procedures to follow would be as outlined previously, with special consideration for a sex-linked trait.

REFERENCES

Brand, E., and G. F. Cahill. 1936. Canine cystinuria. III. J. Biol. Chem. 15:114.
Brand, E., G. F. Cahill, and B. Kassell. 1940. Canine cystinuria. V. Family history of two cystinuric dogs and cystine determinations in dog urine. J. Biol. Chem. 133:431–36.
Bovee, K. C., and S. Segal. 1971. Canine cystinuria and cystine calculi. The newer knowledge about dogs. Proc. 21st Gaines Vet. Symp.
Finco, D. R. 1974. Congenital and Inherited Renal Diseases: Current Veterinary Therapy. V. Philadelphia, London, Toronto: W. B. Saunders.
Holtzapple, P. G., K. Bovee, C. F. Rea, and S. Segal. 1969. Amino acid uptake by kidney and jejunal tissue from dogs with cystine stones. Science 166:1525–27.
Knox, W. E. 1966. Cystinuria. In The Metabolic Basis of Inherited Disease, 2nd ed. Edited by J. B. Stanbury, J. B. Wyngaarden, and D. S. Frederickson. New York: McGraw-Hill.

FAMILIAL RENAL DISEASE

A chronic renal disease has been detected in the Norwegian elkhound. The disease first became apparent at varying ages (8 months to 5 years). Clinical signs are those of renal insufficiency. Uremic dogs expressed anorexia, depression, weight loss, anemia, and sometimes polydypsia and polyuria. Dwarfing was also observed.

Pathophysiology

Expressed pathologic conditions varied with the stage of the disease. The kidneys were small, white, and firm.

A sharply demarcated area of tubular necrosis arranged in a radial fashion was observed extending through the medulla and cortex. There were scattered areas with fibrinoid deposits in glomerular capillaries and tubular lumens. Chronic changes were characterized by atrophy of tubules, tubular dilation, hyalinization of the glomeruli, and basement membrane thickening or mineralization, or both.

Inheritance and Recommendation

The mode of inheritance was not established.

Without additional knowledge concerning the means of genetic transmission, a recommendation could not be made other than the avoidance of affected dogs and dogs related to an affected dog.

REFERENCES

Finco, D. R. 1976. Familial renal disease in Norwegian elkhound dogs. Physiologic and biochemical examinations. Am. J. Vet. Res. 37:87–91.
Finco, D. R., H. J. Kurtz, D. G. Low, and V. Perman. 1970. Familial renal disease in Norwegian elkhound dogs. JAVMA 156:747–60.

RENAL AGENESIS

Unilateral renal agenesis (the absence of one kidney) has been reported in dogs, with most observed cases being found in the beagle.

If the remaining kidney is functional, no obvious signs would be noted. In one report the incidence of renal agenesis was found to be 1 in 100 in the beagle.

Pathophysiology

The single kidney appears normal in structure and is approximately 1½ to twice the usual size.

Inheritance and Recommendation

In one study beagles showing renal agenesis could be traced to a certain sire, suggesting a genetic pattern. Dysgenesis (lack of or defectively developed tissue) and hypoplasia (small kidney, normal structure) have been reported in dogs. No genetic pattern was given.

Until a definite pattern of inheritance is established, no absolute recommendation can be made. Do not use affected animals or closely related animals in a breeding program.

REFERENCES

Finco, D. R., et al. 1970. Familial renal disease in Norwegian elkhound dogs. JAVMA 156:747–60.

Fox, M. W. 1964. Inherited polycystic mononephrosis in the dog. J. Hered. 55:29–30.

Kaufmann, C. F., R. F. Soltys, and J. F. Tasker. 1969. Renal cortical hypoplasia with secondary hyperparathyroidism in the dog. JAVMA 155:1679–85.

Krook, L. 1957. The pathology of renal cortical hypoplasia in the dog. Nord. Vet. Med. 9:161–76.

Murti, G. S. 1965. Agenesis and dysgenesis of the canine kidneys. JAVMA 146:1120–24.

Persson, F., S. Persson, and A. Asheim. 1961. Renal cortical hypoplasia in dogs. A clinical study on uraemia and secondary hypoparathyroidism. Acta Vet. Scand. 2:68–84.

Robbins, G. R. 1965. Unilateral renal agenesis in the beagle. Vet. Rec. 77:1345–47.

Vymetal, F. 1965. Case reports: Renal aplasia in beagles. Vet. Rec. 77:1344–45.

CHAPTER 18

Skin

BLACK HAIR FOLLICULAR DYSPLASIA

A heritable appendageal dysplasia has been observed in black and white crossbred littermates. Visible alterations are strictly confined to black hair coat regions. Other regions of the hair coat appear normal. Abnormalities include hypotrichosis, fractured stubby hair lacking sheen, and periodic scaliness of the skin.

Pathophysiology

In affected black hair coat regions, there are irregular distortions and bridges of hair follicle walls and keratinous blockage of the pilary canals. It was suggested that a derangement of the neural crest derivatives was responsible for this condition.

Inheritance and Recommendation

Although affected dogs produced pups in a manner suggesting an inherited trait, numbers were not sufficient to suggest mode of inheritance.

Since the condition appears rare, avoid use of affected and related animals.

REFERENCE

Selmanowitz, V. J., K. M. Kramer, and O. Orentreich. 1972. Canine hereditary black hair follicular dysplasia. J. Hered. 63:43-44.

BLUE DOG SYNDROME

Chronic papillary dermatitis (inflammation of the skin) accompanied by alopecia (hair loss) is observed in blue-colored dogs of various breeds, such as Doberman, Great Dane, whippet, dachshund, etc.

The condition is believed to be genetically induced. The skin condition occurs only on the areas where the coat is blue in color; other areas appear normal. The affected area shows varying degrees of hyperkeratosis (cornified), manifested by generalized scales. One may also observe a disorder of the sebaceous-apocrine glands with a resultant secretion having a disagreeable odor. This type of skin condition may lead to other secondary conditions.

Pathophysiology

The condition resembles a mild follicular pyoderma. Dermatologic signs suggest immune complex disorder (ICD). Pathologic studies have suggested hypoplasia and degeneration of the adrenal cortex with a resultant adrenal cortisol insufficiency.

Inheritance and Recommendation

Genetic predisposition to ICD may predispose certain dogs to immunologic diseases in general rather than to one particular condition. In this case it would appear that the genetic condition for blue coat may be in some way linked, and that blue hair area is more sensitive.

The mode of inheritance for such a condition being multiple at present no recommendation can be made. Those desiring the blue color should be made aware of the possible problem. Select for breeding blue dogs free from the condition.

REFERENCES

Austin, V. H. 1975. Blue dog syndrome. Mod. Vet. Pract. 56(1):34.
Plechner, A. J., and M. S. Shannon. 1977. Genetic transfer of immunologic disorders in dogs. Mod. Vet. Pract. 58(4):341.
_____. 1976. Canine immune complex diseases. Mod. Vet. Pract. 57(11):917–20.

ECTODERMAL DEFECT

Ectodermal conditions resulting in extensive alopecia (lack of hair) have been reported in whippets, cocker spaniels, and miniature poodles. Pups were born exhibiting the condition. The pattern of alopecia was bilaterally symmetrical and included about two-thirds of the body, head, ventral trunk, dorsal pelvic region, and proximal portions of the limbs. At times a reddish scaliness and other clinical skin lesions (graying of skin) were noted.

Pathophysiology

In the alopecic area there is a distinctive absence of hair follicles, erector pili muscles, sebaceous glands, and sweat glands.

Inheritance and Recommendation

Based on such limited data one could not suggest a mode of inheritance, but in the cases reported the condition did occur only in males.

No sound recommendation could be made from such limited data.

REFERENCE

Selmanowitz, V. J., K. M. Kramer, and N. Orentreich. 1970. Congenital ectodermal defect in miniature poodles. J. Hered. 61:196 99.

HYPOTRICHOSIS (HAIRLESSNESS)

Congenital alopecia is basically a condition of reduced amount or absence of hair over areas of the dog's body where hair is normally found. Congenital hairlessness has been reported in miniature poodles and in one case a whippet. Affected animals are usually males. Loss of hair was first observed at about 5 weeks of age. Affected pups had dry, dull, coarse coats, with hair loss initially on the ear, nose, and tail. The condition was progressive over the remainder of the body.

Pathophysiology

Microscopic examination of the affected area of skin (ear) revealed slight hyperkeratosis. Hair covering was sparse, but hair follicles were present. Large accumulations of soft keratin were found mixed with melanin in the hair canals. Heavy accumulations of melanin were in the keratogenous zones and in bulbs of the hair follicles, as well as in many macrophages in the perifollicular stroma. Most cells were prominent in the perivascular sites. Slight hyperkeratosis was found in the axillary skin, along with clusters of normal hair follicles and hairs. Melanin was concentrated in the hair bulbs.

Skin over the dorsolateral lumbar region was slightly hyperkeratotic. Hair follicles were mostly inactive. Hair canals contained soft keratin and melanin.

Inheritance and Recommendation

The close relationship of the affected pups suggests some type of inheritance. Since the trait was observed only in males of one color, the trait could be sex-linked or limited and related to color. Too few dogs are involved for conclusive evidence as to possible inheritance.

With only limited data given on the possible mode of inheritance, the only recommendation would be to avoid the use of affected and related animals in a breeding kennel.

REFERENCES

Conroy, J. D. 1968. Alopecia of dogs and cats. JAAHA 4:200–269.

Conroy, J. D., B. A. Rasmusen, and E. Small. 1975. Hypotrichosis in miniature poodle siblings. JAVMA 166:697–99.

Selmanowitz, V. J., K. M. Kramer, and N. Orentreich. 1970. Congenital ectodermal defect in miniature poodles. J. Hered. 61:196–99.

———. 1972. Canine hereditary black hair follicular dysplasia. J. Hered. 63:43–44.

Thomsett, L. R. 1961. Congenital hypotrichia in the dog. Vet. Rec. 73:915–17.

CHAPTER 19

Other Structures

CALCINOSIS CIRCUMSCRIPTA (CALCIUM GOUT)

Calcinosis circumscripta refers to granulomatous lesions (nodules) that are primarily calcium salts circumscribed by fibrous tissue. The condition is found mostly in the large breeds of dogs such as the German shepherd (highest incidence), Irish wolfhound, pointer, boxer, Great Dane, bull terrier, greyhound, Labrador, dachshund, beagle, Sealyham, and Norwich staghound. The incidence is highest in dogs up to 2 years of age but this condition does occur in older animals.

The lesions appear as firm, painless nodules in the subcutaneous tissue, most often on the limbs, and occur especially on the tarsus, foot, and elbow, as well as in other locations (skin, vertebra, etc.). The average size of the nodules is 1½ to 3 cm in diameter, but some may reach 10 cm. The lesion may grow slowly. In some cases the skin above the nodules ulcerates and one observes a chalky, puttylike, white fluid discharge.

Pathophysiology

The lesion is a subcutaneous tumorlike mass that may be closely adherent to underlying bony or tendinous structures or to the skin itself. Tumors may be single or multiple in the same area, or multiple and diffuse. Lesions are attached to underlying structures.

Histologic lesions have been summarized as discrete areas of mineralized material in an apparently mucinous matrix, surrounded by a zone of granulation tissue consisting mainly of histiocytes and foreign

177

body giant cells. Differences are found among some lesions. Calcinosis circumscripta involving the feet has been reported only in dogs with renal disease. This relationship could involve alterations of calcium and phosphorus.

Inheritance and Recommendation

The exact cause of the condition is not known. Trauma may be involved. However, the condition is usually restricted to large breeds. Also it is found in closely related animals. It would appear that there is some heritable basis for the development of the lesion.

No genetic recommendation can be made without more information.

REFERENCES

Christie, G. S., and A. G. Jabara. 1964. Apocrine cystic calcinosis and the sweat gland origin of calcinosis circumscripta in the dog. Res. Vet. Sci. 5:317–22.

Cotchin, E. 1960. Calcium gout (kalkgicht) and calcinosis circumscripta in dogs. Br. Vet. J. 116:3–8.

Douglas, S. W., and D. F. Kelly. 1966. Calcinosis circumscripta of the tongue. J. Small Anim. Pract. 7:441–43.

Filo, G. L., and H. Tvedten. 1975. Cervical calcinosis circumscripta in three related Great Dane dogs. JAAHA 11:507–10.

Legendre, A. M., and A. W. Dade. 1974. Calcinosis circumscripta in a dog. JAVMA 164:1192–94.

Owen, L. N. 1967. Calcinosis circumscripta (calcium gout) in related Irish wolfhounds. J. Small Anim. Pract. 8:291–92.

Seawright, A. A., and L. R. Grono. 1961. Calcinosis circumscripta in dogs. Aust. Vet. J. 37:421–25.

Thompson, S. W., D. J. Sullivan, and R. A. Pedersen. 1959. Calcinosis circumscripta: A histochemical study of the lesions in man, dogs, and a monkey. Cornell Vet. 49:265–85.

Vaughn, L. C. 1962. The radiographic features of calcinosis circumscripta (kalkgicht, calcium gout) in the dog. Vet. Rec. 74:988–89.

_____. 1967. B.S.A.V.A. Orthopoedic Group. J. Small Anim. Pract. 8:649–53.

LARYNGEAL-TRACHEAL COLLAPSE

Laryngeal problems (laryngeal collapse) are most common in brachycephalic dogs. One observes difficult respiration, mouth breathing, snoring sounds, etc. Respiratory distress is usually progressive in nature.

Collapsed trachea is reported to be more common in the toy breeds. Tracheal collapse results in both inspiratory and expiratory distress that increases following excitement or exercise. In severe cases, a loud, honking cough accompanies expiration. Secondary cardiac conditions may develop.

Pathophysiology

Laryngeal collapse results from a negative pressure or partial vacuum created during inspiration due to stenotic nares, elongation of the soft palate, or a combination of the two. First, one finds an eversion of the lateral laryngeal ventricles. During inspiration the soft palate is drawn into the lumen of the larynx. This makes inspiration more difficult and increases the negative pressure. Eventually the larynx is altered due to the negative pressure, and the soft mucosal lining of the lateral ventricles (wall of larynx) evert. The everted tissue adds to the already partially obstructed passageway and results in an additional increase in negative pressure. The cuneiform tubercles of the arytenoid cartilage lose their rigidity and are drawn into the laryngeal lumen, with still further obstruction. The cuneiform tubercles may fold or collapse.

The actual cause of the trachea collapse is not well documented, but a demineralization of the cartilaginous rings occurs, with a resultant loss of rigidity. The trachea is soft and flaccid.

Inheritance and Recommendation

A definite genetic pattern for the collapse of the trachea (when and if inherited) and for the laryngeal problems outlined is not given in the literature. Laryngeal problems may be in many cases secondary to and result from the abnormal anatomic structures observed in some breeds. These structures are under genetic control.

Avoid the use of affected individuals in a breeding program, and use close relatives initially with caution. For those breeds where abnormal structure is selected for, choose animals for breeding that show fewer respiratory disorders.

REFERENCES

Leonard, H. C. 1960. Collapse of the larynx and adjacent structures in the dog. JAVMA 137:360-64.
_____. 1971. Surgical correction of collapsed trachea in dogs. JAVMA 158:598-600.

PART III

Abnormalities of the Cat

Section A:

DEFECTS WITH A PROBABLE GENETIC BASE

CHAPTER 20

Cardiovascular System

PATENT DUCTUS ARTERIOSUS

Patent ductus arteriosus is one of the most common shunting lesions in the cat and involves certain valvular anomalies and septal defects. In this defect there is a nonclosure of the ductus arteriosus postnatally with a left to right shunt. A small defect results in the shunting of blood so that an enlargement of the left ventricle occurs. Auscultation reveals a continuous murmur over the pulmonic area. The smaller the duct the louder the murmur and the longer it lasts. Radiographs of the thorax reveal an enlarged round cardiac silhouette and fluid-filled lungs. An electrocardiogram shows left ventricular and atrial hypertrophy. The defect is usually accompanied by an increased oxygen tension in the pulmonary artery and normal heart pressures unless pulmonary hypertension develops. The animal will remain acyanotic until pulmonary hypertension occurs, and when it does occur exercise or stress may cause cyanosis. The condition is easily detected and can be corrected surgically.

Inheritance and Recommendation

This defect shows a possible genetic cause. In one study two Siamese kittens from the same litter were affected. In another litter, two of three kittens sired by a male with patent ductus were affected. The mode of inheritance is not certain, however.

Do not use affected animals or their close relatives for breeding purposes.

REFERENCES

Cohen, J. S., L. P. Tilley, S. Liu, and W. D. DeHoff. 1975. Patent ductus arteriosis in five cats. JAAHA 11:95–101.
Linde-Sipman, J. S. van de; T.S.G.A.M. van den Ingh; and J. P. Koeman. 1973. Congenital heart abnormalities in the cat: A description of sixteen cases. Zentralbl. Veterinaermed. A. 20:419–25.
Perkins, R. L. 1972. Multiple congenital cardiovascular anomalies in a kitten. JAVMA 160:1430–31.
Severin, G. A. 1967. Congenital and acquired heart disease. JAVMA 151:1733–36.

ENDOCARDIAL FIBROELASTOSIS

Endocardial fibroelastosis was originally called fetal carditis because it was thought to be due to an intrauterine infection. Its supposed infectious origin is now rather doubtful so it has been given the descriptive name of endocardial fibroelastosis. The occurrence of the defect is common in humans but uncommon in cats. Affected kittens appear normal at birth but mature slowly, stop nursing, become quiet, and die after a short illness.

Necropsy often reveals severe dehydration, pulmonary edema, and cardiac dilation and hypertrophy. The dilation and hypertrophy of the left ventrical are usually the most extreme, with the endocardium being thickened and opaque, obscuring the normal muscular markings. Partial aortic stenosis may also be present.

Microscopic examination often reveals fibroelastosis of the endocardium as well as myocardial hypertrophy.

Inheritance and Recommendation

Evidence suggests that this defect may have a hereditary basis but this has not been proved. The defect appears to be most common in the Siamese breed.

Parents of affected kittens and other close relatives should not be used for breeding.

REFERENCES

Anderson, R. H., and J. Kelly. 1956. Endocardial fibroelastosis. I. Endocardial fibroelastosis associated with congenital malformations of the heart. Pediatrics 18:513–38.
Bohn, F. K., J. W. Buchanan, and D. F. Kelly. 1970. Pathologic conference case presentation. JAVMA 157:1360–77.
Eliot, T. S., F. P. Eliot, C. C. Lushbaugh, and V. T. Slager. 1958. First report of the occurrence of neonatal endocardial fibroelastosis in cats and dogs. JAVMA 133:271–74.
Linde-Sipman, J. S. van de; T.S.G.A.M. van den Ingh; and J. P. Keoman. 1973. Congenital heart abnormalities in the cat: A description of sixteen cases. Zentralbl. Veterinaermed. A. 20:419–25.

CHAPTER 21

Sensory Organs

ABNORMAL VISUAL PATHWAYS

Siamese cats—along with white tigers, pearl mink, and albino rats—have certain genetic anomalies in which reduced pigmentation is associated with a congenital abnormality of the central visual pathways. This abnormality may be associated with crossed and squinted eyes. The abnormality of the visual pathways has been found in all Siamese cats examined.

Pathophysiology

The light color of Siamese cats is a temperature-sensitive variant of the gene that causes albinism. The coat color is pale except for body extremities. The eyes are blue rather than lacking pigment as in the true albino, which has pink eyes.

All abnormalities observed are present at birth. Studies show that this condition is a result of an abnormal organization within the major retinal pathways. The crossed and squinted eyes appear to be due to the improper control of the eye muscles and therefore appear to be defects of the oculomotor system.

Inheritance and Recommendation

Because the abnormal vision is congenital, it appears to have a genetic cause. It appears that the gene responsible for this kind of albinism also affects the visual pathways in fetal development. Since so many species of albino animals have the same ocular defect, probably one pair of genes with pleiotrophic effects rather than two closely linked genes, produces albinism and the ocular defect.

185

It does not appear that one can breed pure Siamese cats without the occurrence of these defects.

REFERENCES

Guillery, R. W. 1974. Visual pathways in albinos. Sci. Am. 230:44–54.
Kalil, R. E., S. R. Jhaveri, and W. Richards. 1971. Science 174:302–5.

FELINE RETINAL DISEASE

Degeneration of the retina of the eye has been observed in many species. This disease is frequently observed in the Persian cat and in some other breeds as well.

Regardless of the cause, early cases of the disease are characterized by tapetal granularity and retinal vascular thinning. As the disease progresses, there is a marked increase in tapetal reflectivity and loss of retinal vessels to a point where they are completely absent and the cats are blind.

The age of onset of the disease varies with the cause and may be quite variable. In Persian kittens the opthalmoscopic abnormalities are present by 10–12 weeks of age; other cases appear after 6–12 months of age.

Inheritance and Recommendation

In the Persian breed, an autosomal recessive gene is implicated. In other breeds, the mode of inheritance has not been determined, but in some cases autosomal recessive genes may also be involved as well as nongenetic causes.

In cases due to an autosomal recessive gene, affected individuals and their close relatives should not be used for breeding purposes.

REFERENCES

Bellhorn, R. W., and C. A. Fischer. 1970. Feline central retinal degeneration. JAVMA 157:842–49.
Morris, L. M., Jr. 1965. Feline degenerative retinopathy. Cornell Vet. 55:295–308.
Rubin, L. F. 1963. Atrophy of rods and cones in the cat retina. JAVMA 142:1415–20.
Rubin, L. F., and D. Lipton. 1973. Retinal degeneration in kittens. JAVMA 162:467–69.
Scott, P. P., J. P. Greaves, and M. G. Scott. 1964. Nutritional blindness in the cat. Exp. Eye Res. 3:357–64.

DEAFNESS

The correlation between white coat color, blue eyes, and deafness in cats has been known for a long time. Deafness has been observed to be associated with similar conditions in other mammals, including the mouse, dog, and human.

Research has shown that the autosomal dominant gene (W), which has complete penetrance in producing white fur in the cat, also causes blue eyes and deafness in some but not all cats carrying the gene. The dominant gene (W) apparently is not related to true albinism. Blue eyes have been reported to occur in recessive Burmese dilution (c^b) and Siamese dilution (c^s) cats. These are alleles at the C locus, which is considered homologous with albino loci in other species. No unusual incidence of deafness has been reported in such blue-eyed cats.

It has been proposed that homozygous (WW) white cats are more likely to be deaf than are those that are heterozygous (Ww). Matings made among white cats show a positive correlation between blue eyes in the offspring and in their parents. One report suggested that genes controlling blue eyes were independent of those for white fur, but these genes were able to express themselves phenotypically only in the presence of the white gene (W).

In one study, 69 of 162 white cats born were deaf in one or both ears. Only one of 60 pigmented cats tested was deaf.

The syndrome (blue-eyed, white, and deaf) appears to result from a dominant autosomal gene (W) that is fully dominant with complete penetrance for the production of white fur, with incomplete penetrance for deafness, and incomplete dominance for the production of the blue iris. The common pathway of action of the (W) gene appears to be on the development of the structures derived from the neural crest.

Inheritance and Recommendation

Autosomal dominant white genes (W) are involved, with pleiotrophic effects.

In breeding white cats, blue eyes and deafness cannot be avoided in some. To be avoided it would be necessary to breed pigmented cats.

REFERENCES

Bamber, R. C. 1933. Correlation between white coat colour, blue eyes, and deafness in cats. J. Genet. 27:407–13.

Bergsma, D. R., and K. S. Brown. 1971. White fur, blue eyes, and deafness in the domestic cat. J. Hered. 62:171–85.

Bosher, S. K., and C. S. Hallpike. 1965. Observations of the histogenesis of the inner ear degeneration of the deaf white cat. Proc. Royal Soc. B. 162:147–70.

_____. 1966. Observations of the histogenesis of the inner ear degeneration of the deaf white cat and its possible relationship to the aetiology of certain unexplained varieties of human congenital deafness. J. Laryngol. 80:222–35.

Robinson, R. 1959. Genetics of the domestic cat. Bibliog. Genetica 18:273–362.

Whiting, P. W. 1918. Inheritance of coat-color in cats. J. Exp. Biol. 25:539–69.

Whiting, P. W. 1919. Inheritance of white-spotting and other color characteristics in cats. Am. Nat. 53:473–82.

Whitehead, J. E. 1965. Inheritance pattern of deafness in white-coated cats. Mod. Vet. Pract. 46(4):28.

Wilson, T. G., and F. Kane. 1959. Congenital deafness in white cats. Acta Oto-Laryngol. 50:269–77.

Wolff, D. 1942. Three generations of deaf white cats. J. Hered. 33:39–43.

FOLDED EARS

The condition of folded ears is known by cat fanciers as "fold-ear" cats. These cats have entrancing faces and are greatly admired by cat lovers. The condition in some individuals is associated with skeletal abnormalities of the tail and lower extremities. The most obvious skeletal defect is a short, stumpy tail about 5½ inches long, which is due to a shortening of the coccygeal vertebrae. Affected cats and kittens walk slowly with a hobbling gait and tend to stop and lie down on one flank. Frequently there is an overgrowth of the claws, which curl around and penetrate the foot pads, causing considerable pain.

Inheritance and Recommendation

The condition is assumed to be heritable, but the true mode of inheritance has not been established. The presence of the folded ears alone is thought to be due to the heterozygous condition, whereas the presence of both the folded ears and skeletal lesions is thought to be characteristic of the homozygous animal.

Do not use affected individuals for breeding purposes.

REFERENCES

Jackson, O. F. 1974. A heritable osteodystrophy of the extremities of the cat. Proc. Netherlands Small Anim. Vet. Assoc., p. 21.

———. 1975. Congenital bone lesions in cats with fold-ears. Bull. Feline Advisory Bureau. 14:2–4.

FOUR EARS

The condition of four ears is very rare and involves a small extra pinna on each side of the head. The condition is always bilateral, and microphthalmia and micrognathia are associated with it.

Four ears appear to affect the physiologic activity and temperament of individuals, making them less active and more lethargic, although body size appears to be normal.

Inheritance and Recommendation

This is a simple autosomal recessive trait as shown by mating tests.

Affected individuals and their close relatives should not be used for breeding purposes.

REFERENCE

Little, C. C. 1957. Four-ears: A recessive mutation in the cat. J. Hered. 48:57.

CHAPTER 22

Bones and Joints

SPINA BIFIDA

Most cats possess a long tail, but one breed, the Manx cat, is unusual because it possesses a short or stumpy tail or the tail is completely lacking. The mating of Manx with Manx cats produces a preponderance of tailless cats, but a few have a tail of normal length. Litter size appears to be lower when Manx × Manx matings are made as compared to Manx × tailed or tailed × tailed matings. This suggests that the tailless condition may be at least partially lethal. Further evidence shows that the Manx factor is sometimes accompanied by locomotor abnormalities of the hind limbs and fecal and urinary incontinence.

Pathophysiology

Two Manx kittens with locomotor and fecal and urinary incontinence were studied. Radiologic examination revealed 7 normal lumbar vertebrae, 3 hypoplastic sacral vertebrae, and 3 coccygeal vertebrae in 1 kitten, but only 1 coccygeal vertebra in the other. Further examination revealed abnormalities in some of the lumbar vertebrae and very small sacral segments. Some of the nerves were threadlike and barely traceable. These conditions apparently were responsible for the abnormal side effects of the tailless condition.

Inheritance and Recommendation

The tailless condition appears to be due to an autosomal dominant gene with varied expressivity and possibly incomplete penetrance. Some workers have proposed that individuals without tails are homozygous dominant, whereas those with short or stumpy tails are heterozygous for the dominant tailless gene. However, the tailless condition appears to be more complex than this.

The evidence suggests that it is not possible to breed tailless cats without some abnormal side effects. It is also evident that the tailless condition does not breed true. If the objective is to produce a breed of cats without tails, the fact that some of the progeny produced will have long tails, some short tails and other abnormalities, as well as possible fetal death losses, makes this impossible. The breeder must accept these adversities if he is trying to breed such animals.

REFERENCES

Frye, F. L. 1968. Spina bifida occulta with sacro-coccygeal agenesis in a cat. Anim. Hosp. 3:238–42.

Frye, F. L., and L. L. McFarland. 1965. Spina bifida with raduschisis in a kitten. JAVMA 146:481–82.

James, C. C. M., L. P. Lassman, and B. E. Tomlison. 1969. Congenital anomalies of the lower spine and spinal cord in Manx cats. J. Pathol. 97(2):269–76.

Kitchen, H., R. E. Murray, and B. Y. Cockrell. 1972. Animal model for human disease in Manx cats. Am. J. Pathol. 68:203–6.

Leipold, H. W., K. Huston, B. Blauch, and M. M. Guffy. 1974. Congenital defects of the caudal vertebral column and spinal cord in Manx cats. JAVMA 164:520–23.

Martin, A. H. 1971. A congenital defect in the spinal cord of the Manx cat. Vet. Pathol. 8:232–38.

Todd, N. B. 1961. The inheritance of taillessness in Manx cats. J. Hered. 52:228–32.

_____. 1964. The Manx factor in domestic cats. J. Hered. 55:225–30.

POLYDACTYLISM

The cat normally has four digits on each hind foot and five on each front foot, but cats with more than the normal 18 digits are not uncommon. The number of extra digits in cats is quite variable. The trait is found in both sexes.

Inheritance and Recommendation

Polydactylism appears to be due to an autosomal dominant gene with variable phenotypic expression.

Do not use animals showing the trait for breeding purposes.

REFERENCES

Danforth, C. H. 1947. Heredity of polydactyly in the cat. J. Hered. 38:107–12.

_____. 1947. Morphology of the feet of polydactyly cats. Am. J. Anat. 80:143–71.

Howe, F. A. 1902. A case of abnormality in cat's paw. Am. Nature 36:511–26.

Wilder, B. G. 1868. On a cat with supernumerary digits. Boston Soc. Nat. Hist. 11:3–6.

Sis, R. F., and R. Getty. 1968. Polydactylism in cats. Vet. Med. Small Anim. Clin. (Oct.):948–51.

CHAPTER 23

Neuromuscular System

CEREBELLAR HYPOPLASIA

Cerebellar hypoplasia appears to be common among neonatal cats and has been described in the literature on numerous occasions in the past 20 00 years. It is sometimes called spontaneous ataxia and neuroaxonal dystrophy. It appears to be similar to abnormalities described in humans and some domestic animals. It is possible that this condition is due to more than one basic cause.

Pathophysiology

Symptoms of this disease become evident shortly after birth and are expressed more severely in some individuals than in others. Affected animals are unable to maintain normal posture and equilibrium when standing and show a distinct incoordination of gait. Affected animals overreach with their paws and have a poor placing reflex. As a rule affected animals fall on their side or backward, although forward falls in a somersault manner have been observed. Head bobbing or nodding also occurs. The condition seems to be accentuated when the animals are blindfolded. Sometimes they show a pupillary reflex, and vision appears to be impaired. Upon examination the cerebellum appears to be smaller than normal, with hypoplasia of the granular layer.

In one study, affected kittens were colored similar to the "lilac" color in Siamese cats, but their unaffected littermates were black.

One report indicated that this same condition was a result of an intrauterine or perinatal infection of the young by the virus known as panleukopenia (PLV). The authors induced the condition in kittens by intrauterine infections with PLV, and this virus was isolated from the various organs of affected kittens for considerable periods after birth. This induced condition appeared to be analogous with rubella infections in humans.

Inheritance

Some research workers feel that the condition is inherited and it is possible that inheritance is the basic cause in some instances. In one experiment where affected cats had a coat color similar to the "lilac" color in Siamese cats, evidence suggested that both the abnormal color and the ataxia were inherited as autosomal recessive traits. It could not be determined if each trait was conditioned by two separate pairs of closely linked genes, or if both were caused by pleiotrophic effects of one pair of recessive genes.

Since the condition has also been induced by virus infections, it is likely that it is not always inherited, although the susceptibility to the virus may have a genetic base.

Recommendation

Since not all cases of cerebellar hypoplasia are genetic, discrimination against using affected individuals, their littermates, or their parents for breeding purposes may not always prevent the disease. If such individuals and their close relatives are not used for breeding purposes, the frequency of the inherited condition is reduced. This appears to be the procedure of choice.

REFERENCES

Blood, D. C. 1946. Cerebellar hypoplasia and degeneration in the kitten. Aust. Vet. J. 22:120-21.

Brouwer, B. 1934. Familial olivo-ponto-cerebellar hypoplasia in cats. Psychiatr. en Neurol. Bl. 38:352-67.

Campbell, A. M. G. 1967. Feline and human ataxia. Lancet 2:265-66.

Csiza, C. K. 1970. Feline panleukopenia virus as an etiological agent of ataxia: Pathogenesis and immune carrier state. Cornell Univ. thesis.

Kilham, L., G. Margolis, and E. D. Colby. 1967. Congenital infections of cats and ferrets by feline panleukopenia virus manifested by cerebellar hypoplasia. Lab. Invest. 17:465-80.

Woodard, J. C., G. H. Collins, and J. R. Hessler. 1974. Feline hereditary neuroaxonal dystrophy. Am. J. Pathol. 74:551-56.

FELINE TREMORS

Tremors develop first at approximately 2 weeks of age in the affected kittens. The tremors are fine and fibrillary at first but become progressively more severe and gross until they reach a peak at 7–8 weeks of age. They are intensified by movement or excitation. Four affected cats were raised to adulthood. The tremors were reduced in severity as these cats matured, but clinical signs and behavioral changes were evident.

Changes were observed in the nervous system and skeletal muscle tissue of one affected adult cat. These included neuronal degeneration in the ventral horns of the spinal cord gray matter with gliosis and increased vascularity. Similar changes occurred in motor nuclei of the medulla. Muscle fibers varied in size, with an atrophy and basophilia of sarcoplasm in some fibers.

Inheritance and Recommendation

This is an autosomal recessive trait.

Do not use affected individuals or their close relatives for breeding purposes.

REFERENCE

Hegreberg, G. A. 1973. New inherited disorders of the dog and cat. Western Vet. 12:6–8.

HYDROCEPHALUS

Hydrocephalus consists of an abnormal accumulation of fluid in the ventricles of the brain. The frequency of occurrence is unknown but is probably rare.

Pathophysiology

At necropsy the lateral ventricles of the brain appear dilated. The animal shows no response to external stimuli except to the sight of food. Associated defects include edema of the limbs, harelip, and sometimes cleft palate.

Inheritance and Recommendation

This is possibly an inherited recessive lethal in Siamese cats.

Parents of affected individuals or their littermates should not be used for breeding.

REFERENCES

Jackson, O. F. 1969. Congenital abnormalities in kittens. Vet. Rec. 84:76.
Silson, M., and R. Robison. 1969. Hereditary hydrocephalus in the cat. Vet. Rec. 84:477.

LEUKODYSTROPHY

Leukodystrophy is a neurologic disorder in cats that is accompanied by a progressive deterioration beginning at approximately 2 weeks of age. At first the affected kittens have a peculiar piercing cry, and later they become less aggressive in their competition with littermates during the nursing period. They also develop a progressive ataxia involving the rear limbs. Vision impairment occurs early in the course of the disease, and convulsions have been noted. As neurologic deterioration progresses, opisthotonos and paralysis of the rear limbs develop. Affected kittens die by the age of 5–6 weeks.

Microscopic examination shows a severe demyelinating leukoencephalopathy (degeneration of white matter in the brain). Glial cells are numerous and astrocytes are prominent and enlarged in the areas of severe demyelination. Glial cell cytoplasmic inclusions appear to be glycolipid material.

Inheritance and Recommendation

Inheritance is not definitely determined but this disorder is probably an autosomal recessive trait.

Do not use individuals closely related to affected kittens for breeding purposes.

REFERENCES

Hegreberg, G. A. 1973. New inherited disorders of the dog and cat. Western Vet. 12:6–8.
Johnson, K. H. 1970. Globoid leukodystrophy in the cat. JAVMA 150:2057–67.

NEURONAL G_{M1} GANGLIOSIDOSIS

Neuronal G_{M1} gangliosidosis has been described in both humans and cats. Between 2 and 4 months of age affected cats become weak, make slow gains, and show incoordination of the hind legs and a slight tremor of the limbs and head. Impaired vision and recurring convulsions occur at about 1 year of age.

Pathophysiology

The progressive motor disability appears to be caused by an extensive neuronal degeneration as a result of the accumulation of G_{M1} ganglioside in the cerebral cortex.

Inheritance and Recommendation

The condition is due to an autosomal recessive pair of genes.

Close relatives, especially the parents, should not be used for breeding purposes.

REFERENCES

Baker, H. J., and J. R. Lindsey. 1974. Animal model of human disease: Feline G_{M1} gangliosidosis. Am. J. Pathol. 74:649–52.

Baker, J. J., J. R. Lindsey, G. M. McKhann, and D. F. Farrell. 1971. Neuronal G_{M1} gangliosidosis in a Siamese cat with beta-galactosidase deficiency. Science 174:838–39.

Blakemore, W. F. 1972. G_{M1} gangliosidosis in a cat. J. Comp. Pathol. 82:179–85.

Farrell, D. F., H. J. Baker, R. M. Herndon, J. R. Lindsey, and G. M. McKhann. 1973. Feline G_{M1} gangliosidosis: Biochemical and ultrastructural comparisons with the disease in man. J. Neuropathol. Exp. Neurol. 32:1–18.

CHAPTER 24

Digestive System

ESOPHAGEAL ACHALASIA

Achalasia, or the failure of relaxation of the esophagus, has been reported in cats. Food normally stimulates the muscles of the wall of the esophagus causing contractions that move the food toward the stomach. When achalasia is present, the muscles around the opening to the stomach do not relax and open only when the column of food builds up in the esophagus in large enough quantities to force its way through the opening. In affected cats, vomiting may occur and there are varying degrees of esophageal dilation at different locations. Food is often regurgitated immediatley after eating. Pneumonia, pulmonary abcesses, and chronic sinusitis may result from this defect.

It is not a common defect but has been reported by several research workers.

Inheritance and Recommendation

While not proved, the condition appears to be inherited as an autosomal recessive trait.

Do not use close relatives of defective individuals for breeding.

REFERENCES

Cawley, A. J., and C. L. Gendreau. 1969. Esophageal achalasia in a cat. Can. Vet. J. 10:195.

Clifford, D. H. 1973. Myenteric ganglial cells of the esophagus in cats. Am. J. Vet. Res. 34:1333–36.

Clifford, D. H., F. K. Seifer, C. F. Wilson, E. D. Waddell, and G. L. Guilloud. 1971. Congenital achalasia of the esophagus in four cats of common ancestry. JAVMA 158:1554–60.

HARELIP

Harelip is a congenital deformity of the upper lip in which there is a vertical fissure resembling the cleft upper lip of the hare. It is not common in cats, but its occurrence has been reported. It is sometimes associated with a cleft palate.

Inheritance and Recommendation

Harelip is probably inherited, but the mode of inheritance in cats has not been determined.

Affected animals should not be used for breeding.

REFERENCES

Catcott, E. J. 1964. Feline medicine and surgery. Am. Vet. Publ., Wheaton, Illinois.
Loevy, H. T., and V. L. Fenyes. 1968. Spontaneous cleft palate in a family of Siamese cats. Cleft Palate J. 5:57–60.
Robinson, R. 1971. Genetics for Cat Breeders. Elmsford, N. Y.: Pergamon Press, p. 170.

CHAPTER 25

Endocrine and Metabolic Systems

PORPHYRIA

Porphyria is a metabolic disorder in which excessive amounts of porphyrin are secreted in the urine. Porphyrin is an essential part of the hemoglobin molecule. The condition has been described in several species of animals and in humans, especially in Afrikaners.

In affected individuals, porphyrins accumulate in bones and teeth, giving a brownish discoloration. The urine is also reddish to dark brown and glows red under ultraviolet light.

Inheritance and Recommendation

The condition in cats has been reported to be due to a simple autosomal dominant gene with variable expressivity.

Do not use affected individuals for breeding.

REFERENCES

Glenn, B. L. 1970. Feline porphyria. Comp. Pathol. Bull. 2:2–3.
Glenn, B. L., H. A. Glenn, and I. T. Omtvedt. 1958. Congenital porphyria in the domestic cat (*Felis catus*): Preliminary investigation on inheritance pattern. Am. J. Vet. Res. 29:1653–57.
Tobias, G. 1964. Congenital porphyria in a cat. JAVMA 145:462–63.

CHAPTER 26

Urogenital System

MANX CATS

The Manx breed of cats is thought to have originated on the Isle of Man. The breed possesses a variety of biologic and morphologic characteristics, especially the absence of the tail, which easily distinguishes it from other breeds. The common characteristics of the Manx cat besides the absence of the tail include disproportionally long hind legs, short back, large round head, round-shaped rump, and a rabbity humpy gait. Manx cats showing these characteristics must be completely tailless.

Manx × Manx matings give some kittens with normal-length tails; some with short tails called "stumpies"; others called "high-risers," which have only a mere remnant of cartilaginous material where the tail should be; and the tailless "rumpies," which completely lack coccygeal vertebrae. Some Manx cats develop into show animals and good pets without any other undesirable characteristics besides those mentioned. The Manx breeder, however, finds that a fairly large percentage of the kittens he produces suffers from severe congenital abnormalities that are largely due to spinal lesions. These have to be culled or destroyed. Since litter size in Manx × Manx matings is smaller than normal, the gene may be lethal to some individuals during fetal life.

Inheritance and Recommendation

An autosomal dominant gene is involved, but the inheritance may be quite complex. Certainly the gene varies in its phenotypic expression.

The breeder of Manx cats must be prepared to accept losses before birth and after birth associated with defects that accompany the tailless condition. The elimination of the trait is relatively simple since it is necessary to mate only cats with normal tail length to solve the problem.

REFERENCES

Howell, J. M. 1963. Phenotypic variability of taillessness in Manx cats. J. Hered. 54:165.
James, C. C. M., L. P. Lassman, and B. E. Tomlinson. 1969. Spinal anomalies in Manx cats. J. Pathol. 97:269.
Kerruish, D. W. 1964. The Manx cat and spina bifida. J. Cat Genet. 1:16.
Leipold, H. W., K. Huston, B. Blauch, and M. M. Guffy. 1974. Congenital defects of the caudal vertebrae column and spinal cord in Manx cats. JAVMA 164:520–23.
Martin, A. 1971. A congenital defect in the spinal cord of the Manx cat. Vet. Pathol. 8:232.
Todd, N. B. 1961. The inheritance of tailless Manx cats. J. Hered. 52:228.
_____. 1964. The Manx factor in domestic cats. J. Hered. 55:225.

CRYPTORCHIDISM

Cryptorchidism is the defect in which one or both testicles are retained in the abdominal cavity, in the inguinal canal, or in the inguinal ring. Such testicles are small and atrophied. Unilateral cryptorchids occur more frequently than bilateral cryptorchids.

Inheritance and Recommendation

The condition has been reported to be a simple recessive inherited trait, but it may be more complex.

Even if the condition is corrected by surgery, affected animals and their close relatives should not be used for breeding.

REFERENCE

Catcott, F. J. 1964. Feline medicine and surgery. Am. Vet. Publ., Wheaton, Illinois.

"REX" MUTANT

In "rex" cats the hair of the kittens is wavy and wooly in appearance. In adults the hair is short, plushlike, and curly. Guard hairs and vibrissae are absent or abnormal.

Seven "rex" cats have been studied in detail.

Inheritance and Recommendation

Adequate breeding data have been obtained on four animals. All proved to be due to a simple autosomal recessive gene, but two different loci seemed to be involved. This shows that a similar phenotypic resemblance does not guarantee that only one pair of genes is involved.

Do not use affected individuals or their close relatives for breeding.

REFERENCES

Jude, A. C. 1953. A "rex" mutant in the cat. Nature 172:81–82.
Robinson, R. 1971. The rex mutants of the domestic cat. Genetica 42:466–68.
———. 1972. Oregon rex: A fourth rexoid mutant in the cat. Genetica 43:236–38.
———. 1973. The Canadian hairless or sphinx cat. J. Hered. 64:47–49.
Searle, A. G., and A. C. Jude. 1956. The rex type of coat in the domestic cat. J. Genet. 54:506–12.

TORTOISESHELL (TRICOLORED OR CALICO)

The statement is often made that all tortoiseshell or tricolored cats (T-C for short) are females. This is not true. On rare occasions (about 1 out of 3,000), T-C cats are males but many of them are infertile.

The tortoiseshell color often describes a mixture of black and orange colors blended together rather than in large patches. Orange designates colors ranging from a cream or yellow to a dark orange, sometimes referred to as red. Black is really meant to be nonyellow and may include gray, blue, brown, tabby (striped or brindle coat), and black. Calico, or tricolored cats, possess orange, black, and white hairs, usually with the colors in large patches. Obviously, tortoiseshell and calico colors may be used interchangeably in some instances.

The white color in T-C cats is inherited as an autosomal dominant with possible polygenic modifying genes. The white color affects the pigmented colors necessary only when it may mask them in a large amount of white is present. For this reason, in discussing T-C males, the white color is not included. Only the black and orange colors are considered.

Research indicates that the genes for orange and black colors are carried on the X chromosomes. The gene for orange (O) is dominant to the gene for nonorange (o), whereas the gene for black (B) is dominant to the gene (b) for nonblack. It has been suggested that the black gene (B) is an allele of the orange gene (O), but neither is dominant to the other. If this is correct, the following gene combinations would be possible in the female cat:

$$X_B X_B \text{ or } X_B X_b \ldots \ldots \ldots \text{ black}$$
$$X_B X_O \ldots \ldots \ldots \text{ tortoiseshell or}$$
$$\text{calico}$$
$$X_O X_O \text{ or } X_O X_o \ldots \ldots \ldots \text{ orange}$$

It has also been suggested that the genes for black (B) are located on the autosomes rather than on the X chromosome. If true, the orange gene (O) carried on the X chromosome may mask the effect of the black gene (B) carried on the autosomes, which means that orange is epistatic to black.

The spots of orange on the black background may be due to the inactivity of one of the X chromosomes in the cells that produce the orange coat color, according to the Lyon hypothesis. The inactive X chromosome would not be the same in all cells of an individual, but one of the X chromosomes would be inactive (at random) in the various cells. Thus in an individual that possesses genes for black color but is of genetic composition X_oX_o, some of the cells producing coat color would possess the orange gene (O) and they would produce an orange spot on the nonorange or black background. Individuals possessing the nonorange gene (o) would produce fur that was black.

A T-C cat, therefore, should possess two X chromosomes to be this color and would, therefore, be females since females are XX and males XY. A probable explanation of T-C males is that they have a chromosome composition of X_oX_BY, which means they have an extra X chromosome. This may be the explanation of why many T-C males are infertile.

It has been found that about one-third of all T-C male cats are fertile. Some chromosome studies of the T-C cat show that some T-C males are chimeric, or they possess chromosome complements from two genetic sources or two different fertilized eggs. If the cells from such an individual that produced the coat colors possessed two X chromosomes (X_oX_B), the fur would be T-C, but if the cells that produced the sperm cells were XY, it is possible normal fertility would occur. This would be the same thing as a fertilized egg carrying X_oX_B fusing with a fertilized egg carrying X_oY or X_BY chromosomes.

REFERENCES

Bamber, R. C., and E. C. Herdman. 1927. The inheritance of black, yellow and tortoiseshell coat-color in cats. J. Genet. 18:87–97.

Chu, E. H. Y., H. C. Thuline, and D. E. Norby. 1964. Triploid-diploid in a male tortoiseshell cat. Cytogenetics 3:1–18.

Cutler, D. W., and L. Doncaster. 1915. On sterility of the tortoiseshell tomcat. J. Genet. 5:65–73.

Doncaster, L. 1904. On the inheritance of tortoiseshell and related colours in cats. Proc. Cambridge Phil. Soc. 13:35–38.

_____. 1920. The tortoiseshell tomcat: A suggestion. J. Genet. 9:335–37.

Fasnacht, D. E. 1972. A fertile male calico cat. Feline Pract. 2:30–32.

Gregson, N. M., and J. Ishmael. 1971. Diploid-triploid chimerism in 3 tortoiseshell cats. Res. Vet. Sci. 12:275–79.

Ishihara, T. 1956. Cytological studies on tortoiseshell male cats. Cytologia 21:391–98.

Jones, T. C. 1969. Anomalies of sex chromosomes in tortoiseshell male cats. In Comparative Mammalian Cytogenetics, edited by K. Benirschke. New York: Springer-Verlag, pp. 414–33.

Komai, T. 1952. On the origin of the tortoiseshell cat: A correction. Proc. Jap. Acad. 28:150–55.

Little, C. C. 1919. Colour inheritance in cats, with special reference to the colours, black, yellow and tortoiseshell. J. Genet. 8:279–90.

Loughman, M. S., F. L. Frye, and T. B. Condon. 1970. XY/XXY bone marrow mosaicism in three tricolor cats. Am. J. Vet. Res. 31:307–14.

Loughman, W. D., and F. L. Frye. 1974. XY/XXY bone marrow karyotype in a male Siamese crossbred cat. Vet. Med. Small Anim. Clin. 69:1007–11.

Lyon, M. F. 1962. Sex chromatin and gene action in mammalian X-chromosome. Am. J. Hum. Genet. 14:135–48.

Malouf, N. K., K. Benirschke, and D. Hoefnagel. 1967. XX/XY chimerism in a tricolored male cat. Cytogenetics 6:228–41

Matano, J. 1963. A study of the chromosomes in the cat. Jap. J. Genet. 38:147–56.

Pyle, R. L., D. F. Patterson, W. C. D. Hare, D. F. Kelly, and T. Digivlio. 1971. XXY sex chromosome constitution in a Himalayan cat with tortoiseshell points. J. Hered. 62:220–22.

Ramberg, R. E., D. E. Norby, and H. C. Thuline. 1969. Chromosome mosaicism in male calico cats. Northwest Sci. 43:42.

Sprague, L. M., and C. Stormont. 1956. A reanalysis of the problem of the male tortoiseshell cat. J. Hered. 47:237–40.

Thuline, H. C. 1964. Male tortoiseshells, chimerism, and true hermaphroditism. J. Cat Genet. 4:2–3.

Thuline, H. C., and D. E. Norby. 1961. Spontaneous occurrence of chromosome abnormality in cats. Science 134:554–55.

CHAPTER 27

Skin

HAIRLESSNESS

Affected cats have a small amount of hair at birth but this is lost by 2 weeks of age. It is regrown again by 6 weeks and then lost almost completely by the age of 6 months. Only two types of hair are present. These include guard hairs and thinner hairs, which may be either dawn or down hairs. Guard hairs are curved and irregular in diameter.

Close examination shows sparse hairs of deficient types and size in the adult. The hairs are easily dislodged and the hair bulbs are not well formed. The skin is thicker than normal.

Forms of hairlessness in cats have been described in several countries of the world. The occurrence of hairless cats in the United States has resulted in a breed name of "sphinx" cats.

Inheritance and Recommendation

Probably all reported types are autosomal recessives. When hairless cats are mated, they produce only hairless kittens.

To select against the trait do not use hairless cats or their close relatives for breeding purposes.

REFERENCES

Letard, E. 1938. Hairless Siamese cats. J. Hered. 29:173–75.
Robinson, R. 1973. The Canadian hairless or sphinx cat. J. Hered. 64:47–49.
Sternberger, H. 1937. Nonesuch has a birthday—and kittens. J. Hered. 28:310.
_____. 1973. A "cat-dog" from North Carolina. J. Hered. 28:115–16.

CHAPTER 28

Other Structures

DIAPHRAGMATIC HERNIA

Diaphragmatic hernia occurs in about 1 in 1,000 births in cats. The hernia is due to the failure of normal development of all or a part of the diaphragm with part of the abdominal contents extending into the thorax. The pericardial cavity is also expanded, and a pericardial hernia may also be present.

Affected individuals show labored breathing and a double pumping of the abdominal muscles. Respiratory sounds may be absent in the thorax, especially in the right side. The condition may be corrected by surgery.

Inheritance and Recommendation

The condition appears to be inherited as a simple autosomal recessive.

Affected individuals and their close relatives should not be used for breeding purposes.

REFERENCES

Atkins, C. E. 1974. Suspect congenital peritoneopericardial diaphragmatic hernia in an adult cat. JAVMA 165:175–76.

Barrett, R. B., and J. E. Kittrell. 1966. Congenital peritoneopericardial diaphragmatic hernia in the cat. J. Am. Vet. Radiol. Soc. 7:21–26.

Catcott, E. J. 1964. Feline medicine and surgery. Am. Vet. Publ., Wheaton, Illinois.

Frye, F. L., and D. Taylor. 1968. Pericardial and diaphragmatic defects in a cat. JAVMA 152:1507–10.

Jackson, O. F. 1969. Congenital abnormalities in kittens. Vet. Rec. 84:76.

Keep, J. M. 1950. Congenital diaphragmatic hernia in a cat. Aust. Vet. J. 26:193–96.

Leighton, T. L., and E. P. Steffy. 1972. Successful management and repair of diaphragmatic hernia in the cat. Feline Pract. 2:40–43.

Reed, R. A. 1951. Pericardio-peritoneal herniae in mammals with description of a case in the
    domestic cat. Anat. Tech. 110:113–19.

UMBILICAL HERNIA

Umbilical hernia is a fairly common defect in which some of the intestines protrude through the umbilicus into the skin surrounding it, forming a large knot or bump.

Inheritance and Recommendation

The predisposition to the defect in cats is probably inherited, but information is lacking to prove this point. In other species such as cattle and swine, more than one type of umbilical hernia has been described, and different modes of inheritance have been suggested.

Affected individuals and their close relatives should not be used for breeding purposes.

REFERENCES

Hayes, H. M. 1974. Congenital, umbilical and inguinal hernias in cattle, horses, swine, dogs
    and cats: Risk by breed and sex among hospital patients. Am. J. Vet. Res. 35:839–42.
Henricson, B., and S. Bornstein. 1965. Hereditary umbilical hernia in cats. Vet. Bull. 35:453
    (abst.).
Howard, D. R. 1973. Omphalocele in a litter of kittens. Vet. Med. Small Anim. Clin. 68:879.

Section B:

DEFECTS WITH A POSSIBLE GENETIC BASE

CHAPTER 29

Cardiovascular System

TETRALOGY OF FALLOT

Tetralogy of Fallot in humans is a congenital defect that includes multiple anomalies of the heart and associated large vessels. It has been described often in humans and less often in dogs, cattle, and cats. It includes four defects: (1) a ventricular septal defect; (2) pulmonary arterial stenosis; (3) a dextraposition of the aorta; and (4) hypertrophy of the right ventricle of the heart. It is a common cause of cyanosis due to heart disease and is accompanied by retarded growth, intolerance to exercise, and episodes of loss of consciousness (syncope) in affected individuals. Symptoms are the same in cats as in humans. The Blalock-Taussig operation, which increases the pulmonary blood flow by shunting blood from the left side of the heart and diverting it to the pulmonary trunk distal to the pulmonary stenosis, sometimes helps alleviate the condition but tetralogy of Fallot is often fatal.

Inheritance
Unknown.

REFERENCES

Bolton, G. R., S. J. Ettinger, and Si-Kwang Liu. 1972. Tetralogy of Fallot in three cats. JAVMA 160:1622-31.
Bush, M., D. R. Pieroni, D. G. Goodman, R. I. White, V. Thomas, and A. E. James. 1972. Tetralogy of Fallot in a cat. JAVMA 161:1679-86.
Kirby, D., and A. Gillick. 1974. Polycythemia and tetralogy of Fallot in a cat. Can. Vet. J. 15:114-19.

PERSISTENT COMMON ATRIOVENTRICULAR CANAL

Two cats were examined and were found to have a persistent common atrioventricular canal. Both were male domestic short-haired cats about 6 months of age. Both specimens were stunted, emaciated, and lacked stamina. They also showed signs of congestive heart failure. An examination of the heart showed a gross defect in the lowermost part of the interatrial septum and the uppermost part of the interventricular septum. The defects were associated with a cleft mitral valve.

Inheritance

The condition is rare and is not known to be inherited.

REFERENCES

Liu, Si-Kwang, and S. Ettinger. 1968. Persistent common atrioventricular canal in two cats. JAVMA 153:556–62.
Moragules, V. 1943. Persistent common atrioventricular atrium: Report of a case. Arch. Pathol. 25:123–27.

AORTIC STENOSIS

Aortic stenosis is characterized by a narrowing of the aortic orifice or of the aorta. The defect may be supravalvular or subvalvular. The condition may be identified upon examination when there is a harsh systolic ejection murmur on either the right or left side, or a precordial thrill, or an enlarged left ventricle. An anomalous aortic valve may also be present. The condition has been described in several experiments.

Inheritance

Unknown.

REFERENCES

Liu, Si-Kwang. 1968. Supravalvular aortic stenosis with deformity of the aortic valve in a cat. JAVMA 152:55–59.
Severin, G. A. 1967. Congenital and acquired heart disease. JAVMA 151:1733–36.
Tashjian, R. G., K. M. Das, W. E. Palich, R. L. Hamlin, and D. A. Yarns. 1965. Studies on cardiovascular disease in the cat. Ann. N.Y. Acad. Sci. 127:581–605.

PULMONARY STENOSIS

Pulmonary stenosis is an uncommon anomaly in cats in which there is a narrowing of the pulmonary valve at a subvalvular location. Examination showed affected animals had a loud systolic ejection murmur and a precordial thrill at the pulmonic area. The right side of the heart also showed hypertrophy. An aorticopulmonary septal defect is sometimes noted.

Inheritance
Unknown.

REFERENCES
Severin, G. A. 1967. Congenital and acquired heart disease. JAVMA 151:1733–36.
Tashjian, R. J., K. M. Das, W. E. Palich, R. L. Hamlin, and D. A. Yarns. 1965. Studies on cardiovascular disease in the cat. Ann. N.Y. Acad. Sci. 127:581–605.
Will, J. W. 1969. Subvalvular pulmonary stenosis and aorticopulmonary septal defect in the cat. JAVMA 154:913–16.

PERSISTENT RiGHT AORTIC ARCH
Affected kittens often regurgitate their food soon after it is eaten. This may be confirmed radiographically after they consume a semisolid barium meal. The condition is not a common one.

Basically the arch of the aorta develops from the right fourth aortic arch instead of the left. It crosses the esophagus and trachea, forming a vascular ring with the base of the heart, the pulmonary artery, and ligamentum arteriosum, causing esophageal stenosis with dilation proximal to the stricture. It can be corrected surgically by severing the ligamentum arteriosum.

Inheritance
Unknown.

REFERENCES
Buergelt, C. D., P. F. Suter, and W. J. Kay. 1968. Persistent truncus arteriosus in a cat. JAVMA 153:548–52.
Douglas, S. W., R. G. Walker, and M. C. G. Littlewort. 1960. Vet. Rec. 72:91–92.
Hathaway, J. E. 1965. Persistent right aortic arch in a cat. JAVMA 147:255–59.
Jessop, L. 1960. Persistent right aortic arch in the cat causing aesophageal stenosis. Vet. Rec. 72:46.
Reed, J. H., and H. Bonasch. 1962. The surgical correction of a persistent right aortic arch in a cat. JAVMA 140:142–44.
Richmond, B. T. 1968. A case of persistent right aortic arch in the cat. Vet. Rec. 83:169.
Uhrich, S. J. 1963. Report of a persistent right aortic arch and its surgical correction in a cat. J. Small Anim. Pract. 4:337–38.

ATRIAL SEPTAL DEFECT
Defects of the atrial septum occur in cats, but they are rare. If the defects are small, only subclinical changes occur. If they are large, severe

clinical signs and early death may occur. Such defects occur when there is a persistent communication between the left and right atria through the septum primum or foramen ovale. Radiograph examinations reveal an enlarged right ventricle and pulmonary artery as well as pulmonary vascular congestion.

Inheritance
Unknown.

REFERENCES

Linde-Sipman, J. S. van de; T.S.A.G.M. van den Ingh; and J. P. Koeman. 1973. Congenital heart abnormalities in the cat: A description of sixteen cases. Zentralbl. Veterinaermed. A. 20:419–25.
Severin, G. A. 1967. Congenital and acquired heart disease. JAVMA 151:1733–36.

COMMON TRUNCUS ARTERIOSUS
In common truncus arteriosus the aorta, coronary arteries, and the pulmonary artery have a common trunk that is above a defect in the ventricular septum. A funnel chest is sometimes associated with the defect. The defect can usually be identified only at necropsy. It is rare and the cause unknown.

Inheritance
Unknown.

REFERENCES

Buergelt, C. D., P. F. Suter, and W. J. Kay. 1968. Persistent truncus arteriosus in a cat. JAVMA 153:548–51.
Linde-Sipman, J. S. van de; T.S.G.A.M. van den Ingh; and J. P. Koeman. 1973. Congenital heart abnormalities in the cat: A description of sixteen cases. Zentralbl. Veterinaermed. A. 20:419–25.

DEXTRAPOSITION OF THE AORTA
Dextraposition of the aorta is a defect in which there is a displacement of the aorta to the right. It is rare in occurrence and is identified only at necropsy. Other defects associated with it include atresia ani, an enlarged left auricle, a round heart, and absence of ventricular septae and atria.

Inheritance
It is not known if this condition is inherited. It could be due to a virus infection during early intrauterine development.

REFERENCES

Linde-Sipman, J. S. van de; T.S.G.A.M. van den Ingh; and J. P. Koeman. 1973. Congenital heart abnormalities in the cat: A description of sixteen cases. Zentralbl. Veterinaermed. A. 20:419–25.

VENTRICULAR SEPTAL DEFECT

Ventricular septal defect shows a persistent communication between the right and left ventricles of the heart. It is probably a common defect but is seldom diagnosed because most affected kittens die before weaning. Several symptoms help diagnose the condition. Affected individuals usually show labored breathing, a thrill along the sternum, and a pansystolic murmur. Radiographs show an enlarged heart, mainly on the right side. Hydropericardium and an atrial septal defect usually are associated with this defect.

Inheritance

Unknown.

REFERENCES

Linde-Sipman, J. S. van de; T.S.G.A.M. van den Ingh; and J. P. Koeman. 1973. Congenital heart abnormalities in the cat: A description of sixteen cases. Zentralbl. Veterinaermed. A. 20:419–25.
Mann, P. G. H., J. E. Slock, and J. P. Sheridan. 1971. Pulmonary artery banding in the cat: A case report. J. Small Anim. Pract. 12:45–48.
Severin, G. A. 1967. Congenital and acquired heart disease. JAVMA 151:1733–34.

MULTIPLE HEART DEFECTS

A combination of congenital cardiac anomalies was described in a 2-week-old male Siamese kitten. The defects included patent ductus arteriosus, interatrial septal defect, interventricular septal defect, and tricuspid insufficiency. The kitten also had an umbilical hernia. Such cases appear to be quite rare.

The kitten was from a litter of four, two of which were born dead but were not examined. The kitten appeared normal for the first week then lost its appetite and showed signs of weakness and difficult breathing. The kitten was slightly smaller than its surviving littermate and was not as active.

Multiple defects were observed in the heart of a 7-week-old Persian kitten. The kitten was smaller than other members of the same litter and was less vigorous. When examined at 5 weeks of age, a palpable thrill was observed throughout the ventral portion of the thorax and a strong "machinery" murmur was detected by auscultation. Necropsy findings at 7 weeks of age included patent ductus arteriosus, an interatrial septal defect, an interventricular septal defect, and an absence of the aortic and pulmonary valves. It was also noted that the main pulmonary artery and the aorta originated from the wall of the right atrium.

Inheritance

In the first case, whether or not the condition was inherited was not determined, but the sire of the litter died suddenly at 2 years of age. The cause of the sire's death was not determined.

In the second case, whether or not inheritance was involved was not known since only one case was observed.

REFERENCES

Dear, M. G. 1970. An unusual combination of congenital cardiac anomalies in a cat. J. Small Anim. Pract. 11:37–43.

Perkins, R. L. 1972. Multiple congenital cardiovascular anomalies in a kitten. JAVMA 160:1430–31.

SEPTUM MEMBRANACEUM ANEURYSM

Only one case has been described in which necropsy showed that the blind end of the aneurysm (dilation) was under the septal cusp of the tricuspid valve. A dilated left ventricle and a smaller left atrium were also observed.

Inheritance

Unknown.

REFERENCE

Linde-Sipman, J. S. van de; T.S.G.A.M. van den Ingh; and J. P. Koeman. 1973. Congenital heart abnormalities in the cat: A description of sixteen cases. Zentralbl. Veterinaermed. A. 20:419–25.

CHAPTER 30

Sensory Organs

CATARACT

The crystalline lens or lens capsule is opaque in the cataract defect. Nuclear cataract is the commonest type and usually is not progressive. Possible causes of congenital cataracts include intrauterine infections, radiation, prenatal infections of the eye, and heredity. The condition is rare in felines, and little is known about genetic causes.

REFERENCES

Peiffer, R. L., and K. N. Gelatt. 1974. Cataracts in the cat. Feline Pract. 4:34–38.
Preister, W. A. 1972. Congenital ocular defects in cattle, horses, cats, and dogs. JAVMA 160:1504–11.

COLOBOMAS

Colobomas are defects involving fissures in the iris, choroid, or optic nerve. They are rare in occurrence and the cause is unknown.

REFERENCE

Bellhorn, R. W., K. C. Barnett, and P. Henkind. 1971. Ocular colobomas in domestic cats. JAVMA 159:1015–21.

CYCLOPIA

Cyclopia is a congenital defect in which two orbits of the eye are fused into a single cavity containing one rudimentary eye. In the cat it is usually associated with skin and brain anomalies. The condition is rare and the cause is unknown.

REFERENCE

Catcott, E. J. 1964. Feline medicine and surgery. Am. Vet. Publ., Wheaton, Illinois.

ECTOPIC LENS

Ectopic lens is an eye defect in cats in which the lens of the eye is located anteriorly or posteriorly to its normal position. The defect is sometimes accompanied by glaucoma. It is rare in occurrence.

Pathophysiology

The cause appears due to the incomplete development of the suspensory ligaments of the lens or to the degeneration of the zonular fibers.

Inheritance

It is not known if this condition is hereditary.

REFERENCES

Aquirre, C. D., and S. L. Distner. 1973. Microphalda with lentloular lunatlon and sublunatlon in cats. Vet. Med. Small Anim. Clin. 68:498–500.
Catcott, E. J. 1964. Feline medicine and surgery. Am. Vet. Publ., Wheaton, Illinois.

EYELID AGENESIS

Eyelid agenesis is a condition in which the outer one-half of one or both of the eyelids is absent. The tarsus, Meibomian glands, and orbicularis muscles are absent. The eye shows no blink reflex in the portion where the eyelid is missing. Secondary corneal lesions sometimes occur. It is common among Persian cats.

Pathophysiology

The condition appears to be due to the failure of the union of eyelid margins during early embryonic development.

Inheritance

The mode of inheritance is not known.

REFERENCES

Bellhorn, R. W., K. C. Barnett, and P. Henkind. 1971. Ocular colobomas in domestic cats. JAVMA 159:1015–21.
Roberts, S. R., and S. L. Bistner. 1968. Surgical correction of eyelid agenesis. Mod. Vet. Pract. 49:40–43.

CHAPTER 31

Neuromuscular System

MENINGOCELE

Only one case of meningocele is described in the literature. A 4-week-old kitten showed a fluid-filled swelling about 5 cm in diameter on the dorsal portion of the skull.

Pathophysiology

Surgery revealed that the meningocele originated from the junction of the falx cerebri and tentorium cerebelli. The corpus callosu, septum pellucidum, and hippocampal commissure were absent.

Inheritance

Unknown.

REFERENCE

Griffiths, I. R. 1971. Abnormalities in the central nervous system of a kitten. Vet. Rec. 89:123–24.

NUCLEAR JAUNDICE (KERNICTERUS)

Neonatal hyperbilirubinemia of the erythroblastic type has been described in the human and several species of lower animals. A congenital nonhemolytic type of hyperbilirubinemia is rare in humans but has been reported in a strain of rats. A frequent complication of this rare type is kernicterus, or nuclear jaundice. Kernicterus describes a condition in which the bile stains the basal nuclei of the brain, and this may lead to toxic degeneration of the nerve cells, with resulting disabilities. The condition has been described in a kitten. The kitten was one in a litter of four and became ill at the end of the second week. It cried constantly and was reluctant to move for long periods of time. At necropsy, intense yellow discoloration was found in a number of subcortical masses of gray matter. Upon microscopic examination it was found that there was a widespread nerve cell necrosis, with bilirubin staining of some necrotic cells.

Inheritance

Not determined.

REFERENCE

Tryphonas, L., and B. Rozdilsky. 1970. Nuclear jaundice (kernicterus) in a newborn kitten. JAVMA 157:1084–87.

CHAPTER 32

Digestive System

ANODONTIA
One case of anodontia has been reported where a cat showed a complete lack of teeth. This condition is very rare and the cause has not been determined.

REFERENCE

Elzay, R. P., and R. D. Hughes. 1969. Anodontia in a cat. JAVMA 154:667–70.

CLEFT PALATE
Cleft palate, a condition in which there is a median cleft in the palate, has been reported in Siamese cats. Affected kittens are unable to nurse and, when examined, the condition may be diagnosed. The cleft palate condition may be accompanied by the presence of a harelip.

Inheritance and Recommendation
The condition is probably inherited since it appears in certain families. The mode of inheritance is unknown. The chromosome complement of affected kittens is normal.

Affected animals and their close relatives should not be used for breeding.

REFERENCES

Loevy, H. T. 1974. Cytogenic analysis of Siamese cats with cleft palate. J. Dent. Res. 53:453–56.

Loevy, H. T., and V. L. Fenyes. 1968. Spontaneous cleft palate in a family of Siamese cats. Cleft Palate J. 5:57–60.

MEGACOLON

Megacolon is a condition that results in the dilation, elongation, and hypertrophy of the colon of the cat. The myenteric plexus is also absent. Chronic constipation, distention of the abdomen, anorexia, and general malaise are characteristic features. Large masses of fecal material accumulate in the colon. The condition may be corrected surgically by a resection of the gut. The condition is rare and the etiology unknown.

REFERENCE

Yoder, J. T., L. R. Dragstedt, and C. J. Starch. 1968. Partial colectomy for correction of megacolon in a cat. Vet. Med. Small Anim. Clin. 63:1049–52.

CHAPTER 33

Urogenital System

HERMAPHRODITISM

Hermaphroditism is a rare condition in which some of the reproductive organs of both sexes are present in the same individual. In the cat this condition is one in which there is an ovotestis on one side and a testis on the other. It is due to improper differentiation of the gonads in the embryo. It is not known if this condition is inherited. It may be due to an accident of development.

REFERENCES

Bloom, F. 1954. Pathology of the dog and cat. Am. Vet. Publ., Evanston, Illinois.
Harman, M. T. 1917. Another case of gynandromorphism. Anat. Rec. 13:425–35.

HORSESHOE KIDNEY

Horseshoe kidney is due to a symmetrical fusion of the kidneys, usually at the caudal pole and across the midline by means of a thin fibrous cord or band of renal tissue. The fusion occurs early in fetal life and is generally diagnosed radiographically or at necropsy. Vascular abnormalities may also accompany the defect. The occurrence of this defect is not common and the cause is unknown.

REFERENCES

Bloom, F. 1954. Pathology of the dog and cat. Am. Vet. Publ., Evanston, Illinois.
Johnson, C. E. 1914. Pelvic and horseshoe kidneys in the domestic cat. Anat. Anz. 46:69–78.

Story, H. E. 1943. A case of horseshoe kidney and associated vascular anomalies in the domestic cat. Anat. Rec. 86:307–19.

PELVIC KIDNEY

The pelvic kidney is a condition in which the kidney has been displaced to the pelvic region due to an abnormal migration of the precursor of the kidney early in embryonic development. The kidney is also abnormal in shape; vascular abnormalities accompany the condition. The abnormal kidney is subject to hydronephrosis, pyonephrosis, pyelonephritis, and calculi. The abnormal kidney may be mistaken for an abscess, tumor, or some other foreign body when palpated. The condition is rare and the cause unknown.

REFERENCES

Bloom, F. 1954. Pathology of the dog and cat. Am. Vet. Publ., Evanston, Illinois.
Johnson, C. E. 1914. Pelvic and horseshoe kidneys in the domestic cat. Anat. Anz. 46:69–78.

PERSISTENT URACHUS

The urachus is a canal, or tube, within the allantoic stalk that connects the bladder and the umbilicus during embryonic development. After birth it normally loses connection with the umbilicus and is drawn downward toward the bladder. The failure of the allantoic stalk to shrink and stop functioning after birth has been described in the cat. The urachus may be patent and may leak urine outside the body or within the abdominal cavity. It may also remain patent and nonfunctional in later life. The condition is indicated by abdominal distention, but it may be surgically corrected. The liver in affected individuals may be cystic. The condition is rare and the cause is unknown.

REFERENCES

Hansen, J. S. L. 1972. Patent urachus in a cat. Vet. Med. Small Anim. Clin. 67:374–81.
Scherzo, C. S. 1967. Cystic liver and persistent urachus in a cat. JAVMA 151:1329–30.

POLYCYSTIC KIDNEY

In polycystic kidney, multiple cysts replace the renal parenchyma, and they are usually bilateral. The condition is associated with a cystic liver, a cystic pancreas, and perirenal hygroma. Affected individuals have a poor appetite and gradually lose weight. Anemia often occurs and the affected individuals have an abnormal thirst and show polyuria and a terminal uremia. The condition occurs embryologically because of the failure of the collecting tubules of the kidney to unite with the convoluted tubules. The condition is common in occurrence but the cause is unknown.

REFERENCES

Battershell, D., and J. P. Garcia. 1969. Polycystic kidney in a cat. JAVMA 154:665–66.
Bloom, F. 1954. Pathology of the dog and cat. Am. Vet. Publ., Evanston, Illinois.

UNILATERAL FUSED KIDNEY

The fusion occurs in the embryo and is an assymetrical fusion causing the kidneys to appear as a disc or the shape of a dumbbell. The cause of the condition is unknown, and it is rare in occurrence.

REFERENCE

Bloom, F. 1954. Pathology of the dog and cat. Am. Vet. Publ., Evanston, llinois.

UNILATERAL RENAL AGENESIS

Unilateral renal agenesis is the absence of a kidney on one side, usually the right side. The remaining kidney undergoes compensatory hypertrophy. Abnormalities accompanying this defect include uterus unicornis (uterus with one horn), atretic vagina in females, and the absence of the vas deferens in the male. There may be an absence of ureters and renal blood vessels. Unilateral renal agenesis occurs in early embryonic life because of the lack of development of one urogenital ridge. The condition is common and occurs more often in males than in females. It is not known if inheritance is involved.

REFERENCES

Bloom, F. 1954. Pathology of the dog and cat. Am. Vet. Publ., Evanston, Illinois.
Mack, C. O., and J. H. McGlothlin. 1949. Renal agenesis in the female cat. Anat. Rec. 105:445–50.
Reis, R. H. 1966. Unilateral urogenital agenesis with unilateral pregnancy and vascular abnormalities in the cat. Wasmann J. Biol. 24:209–22.

UNILATERAL RENAL HYPOPLASIA

Unilateral renal hypoplasia is a rare defect in which one kidney is small, with reduced parenchyma, and abnormal glomeruli and tubules. Cysts and interstitial fibrosis, or calcification, may also be present. The pelvic ureter and renal blood vessels of the hypoplastic kidney are small and poorly developed. The cause is probably an arrest in the development of the mesonephros in the embryo. It is not known if inheritance is implicated.

REFERENCE

Bloom, F. 1954. Pathology of the dog and cat. Am. Vet. Publ., Evanston, Illinois.

CHAPTER 34

Skin

CUTANEOUS ASTHENIA

Cutaneous asthenia is a rare condition in cats in which the skin is thin, weak, and fragile, and the individual is subject to recurrent lacerations and abscesses. The affected cat becomes emaciated and has pale mucous membranes. The skin is thin and velvety to the touch and is hyperelastic. The condition is accompanied by anemia and enteritis. The dermis and epidermis of the skin are thin and irregular and the dermis is fragmented.

Inheritance and Recommendation

This condition is possibly inherited but the mode is unknown. Affected individuals should not be used for breeding.

REFERENCE

Scott, D. V. 1974. Cutaneous asthenia in a cat resembling Ehler's-Danlos syndrome in man. Vet. Med. Small Anim. Clin. 69:1256-58.

EPITHELIOGENESIS IMPERFECTA

Imperfect skin development in one litter of Siamese kittens has been reported. The condition was accompanied by linear ulcers of the tongue. A histologic examination showed a thinning and the loss of epithelium.

Inheritance

No evidence that heredity was involved was reported, but the same condition has been reported as hereditary in other species such as cattle and sheep.

Affected individuals should not be used for breeding.

REFERENCE

Munday, B. L. 1970. Epitheliogenesis imperfecta in lambs and kittens. Br. Vet. J. 126:47.

CHAPTER 35

Other Structures

PULMONARY TRUNK HYPOPLASIA

Pulmonary trunk hypoplasia is a rare defect in the cat and is due to an extreme reduction in the size of the pulmonary trunk. Clinically it is characterized by difficult breathing. Necropsy reveals an enlarged heart with dilation of the right side. A left rather than a right precava is present.

Inheritance

Unknown.

REFERENCE

Linde-Sipman, J. S. van de; T.S.G.A.M. van den Ingh; and J. P. Koeman. 1973. Congenital heart abnormalities in the cat: A description of sixteen cases. Zentralbl. Veterinaermed. A. 20:419–25.

INTERNAL BRANCHIAL FISTULA

Internal branchial fistula is a rare condition characterized by a fistula that opens into the pharynx and originates from the second branchial arch. There is a sac in the tracheal areas of the lower neck. The cause is unknown.

REFERENCE

Miskowiec, J. F., G. H. Hankes, H. N. Hankes, Jr., and J. E. Bartels. 1974. Internal branchial fistula in a kitten. Vet. Med. Small Anim. Clin. 69:259–63.

INGUINAL HERNIA

Inguinal hernia is a rare defect in which the gut protrudes into the inguinal canal. The cause in cats is unknown, although in some species of animals it is reported to be hereditary.

REFERENCE

Hayes, H. M. 1974. Congenital umbilical and inguinal hernias in cattle, horses, swine, dogs, and cats: Risk by breed and sex among hospital patients. Am. J. Vet. Res. 35:839–42.

PART IV

Abnormalities of the Horse

Section A:

DEFECTS WITH A PROBABLE GENETIC BASE

CHAPTER 36

Hemopoietic and Lymphatic Systems

NASAL BLEEDING

Nasal bleeding has been reported in the English Thoroughbred. The earliest case reported was in a foundation sire, Herod, foaled in 1748. Humorist, who won the English Derby in 1921, died 17 days after the race with this condition. An extensive survey located 185 animals with nasal bleeding, and it was the cause of death in 17.

Pathophysiology

The blood has normal clotting properties in affected individuals so it differs from the hemophilic condition found in dogs and swine. The bleeding is caused by thin, fragile blood vessels that have a tendency to burst under stress. Those blood vessels in the nasal mucosa are the most likely to be affected.

Inheritance and Recommendation

The mode of inheritance appears to be recessive.

This condition is of little importance to the practical breeder because it has been reported only in English Thoroughbreds. It does point out the fact, however, that certain animals that are valuable for one purpose may also possess detrimental genetic factors that lower their value for another. Affected animals and their close relatives should not be used for breeding.

REFERENCES

Robertson, J. B. 1913. The heredity of blood vessel breaking in the Thoroughbred horse. Bloodstock Breed. Rev. 265–71. As reported by F. A. E. Crew and A. D. Buchanan Smith. 1930. The genetics of the horse. Bibliog. Genetica 6:123–70.

Wriedt, C. 1930. Heredity in Livestock. London: Macmillan.

IMMUNODEFICIENCY

A fatal genetic disease that is due to a combined (B- and T-lymphocyte) immunodeficiency in Arabian foals has been reported. Foals suffering from these deficiencies are susceptible to a variety of infections at an early age after the supply of antibodies obtained from the colostrum disappears. The majority of deaths in these foals are due to adenoviral infections.

Pathophysiology

Immunologic responses are mediated by at least two distinct antigen-sensitive lymphocyte populations. Both populations originate from the stem cells in the bone marrow. One population representing 60%–80% of the total lymphocytes in the blood are called T lymphocytes because they appear to undergo maturation in the thymus. The T lymphocytes are responsible for cell-mediated immunity but in the production of some antibodies they cooperate with B lymphocytes. In general the B lymphocytes account for the remainder of the lymphocytes in the blood. The B lymphocytes are distinguished by the presence of immunoglobulin on their surface. In some cases B lymphocytes may be stimulated by T lymphocytes to undergo blast formation leading to the production of antibodies. The lack of the combined action of B and T lymphocytes is the defect described in Arabian foals.

The foals usually receive the normal complement of antibodies from the mother's colostrum, but this type of immunity is passive and the foal later depends on its own antibody production to overcome disease. Some foals die because they do not possess the genetic mechanism to produce the combined B- and T-lymphocyte reaction and thus do not produce the antibodies to fight certain infections.

Inheritance and Recommendation

The condition appears to be an autosomal recessive, which means that two normal carriers of the recessive gene will be expected to produce one out of four foals that have this deficiency.

Affected individuals have very low lymphocyte counts in the blood and there appears to be no detectable immunoglobulin M in the blood of affected foals. The presence of this defect in foals should be determined by the appropriate tests, and the mating of two normal carriers of the defective gene should be avoided.

REFERENCES

McGuire, T. C., and M. J. Poppie. 1973. Hypogammaglobulinemia and thymic hypoplasia in horses:A primary combined immunodeficiency disorder. Infect. Immun. 8:272–77.
_____. 1973. Primary hypogammaglobulinemia and thymic hypoplasia in horses. Fed. Proc. 32:821.

McGuire, T. C., M. J. Poppie, and K. L. Banks. 1974. Combined (B- and T-lymphocyte) immunodeficiency: A fatal genetic disease in Arabian foals. JAVMA 164:70–76.

HEMOPHILIA

Hemophilia is a condition in which the blood does not clot in the normal manner. Several factors are involved in the blood-clotting mechanism, but so-called true or classic hemophilia in the horse is usually considered to be due to a deficiency of factor VIII.

True hemophilia in Thoroughbreds was first described in a foal in Great Britain, and later two hemophilic foals related to the first were found and their blood studied. Three other equine cases of true hemophilia have been described in standard breeds: two in Australia and one in the United States. These cases were observed in male foals unrelated to each other and were not related to those described in Great Britain. Therefore, this condition seems to be quite rare.

Foals appear to be normal at birth but within a few days they develop hematomas on various parts of the body. One foal developed several small hematomas on its back where it had been bitten by its mother.

Laboratory tests show the condition due to a deficiency of factor VIII.

Inheritance

Studies in Great Britain indicate the condition is caused by a sex-linked recessive gene. This is the same mode of inheritance found in humans and dogs.

Recommendation

Because it appears to be a rare condition in horses, it should seldom be encountered in actual practice. If this condition does occur, the mother of the foal is a carrier of the recessive gene and would be expected to transmit the gene to one-half of her offspring; therefore, she should not be used for breeding purposes. Close female relatives such as the affected mare's daughters and her full sisters should also be discriminated against for breeding purposes.

A normal stallion producing an affected foal would not be a carrier of the defective gene because if he possessed it he would be a bleeder. Since he transmits his X chromosome to his daughters and his Y chromosome to his sons he would never transmit this recessive gene to his son.

REFERENCES

Archer, R. K. 1961. True haemophilia (haemophilia A) in a Thoroughbred foal. Vet. Rec. 73:338–40.
Archer, R. K., and B. V. Allen. 1972. True haemophilia in horses. (Letter to the editor.) Vet. Rec. 91:655–56.

Hutchins, D. R., E. E. Lepherd, and I. G. Crook. 1967. A case of equine haemophilia. Aust.
    Vet. J. 43:83–87.
Sanger, V. L., R. E. Mairs, and A. L. Trapp. 1964. Hemophilia in a foal. JAVMA 144:259,

HEMOLYTIC DISEASE

Hemolytic disease is also referred to as hemolytic icterus. It has been observed in foals shortly after birth following the consumption of the colostrum of the mother. It is characterized by a jaundice resulting from the destruction of red blood cells in the peripheral bloodstream. Unlike erythroblastosis fetalis in the human, the foal is not affected at birth, but it has to obtain the antibodies from the colostrum before the jaundice is produced. Death usually follows in a few hours unless the foal is properly treated. Hemolytic disease is relatively rare, however, in horses.

Pathophysiology

Mares that produce icteric foals possess antibodies against the erythrocytes (red blood cells) of the stallions to which they have been mated. If the mare carries a foal with the same antigens in its red blood cells as its sire, she may produce antibodies against these antigens. The mare apparently becomes sensitized when in some manner some of the erythrocytes of the foal or a portion of them enter the bloodstream of the mare. This causes the mare to build antibodies against these antigens. When sensitivity in the mare is great enough, she produces antibodies and secretes them in her colostrum. The foal is born normal, but when it consumes the erythrocyte-destroying antibodies in the colostrum of the mare, its red blood cells are destroyed, it becomes jaundiced, and the blood becomes a light yellow.

The large majority of first hemolytic foals are produced by a mare during her fourth to seventh pregnancies. Once the mare is sensitized against the antigens she is more likely to produce affected foals in later pregnancies. The disease does not occur in every incompatible pregnancy or the frequency of the disease would be much higher than it now appears to be. If the sensitized mare is mated to another stallion whose blood is compatible with hers, the resulting foals may not be affected.

Inheritance

Hemolytic disease has a hereditary basis. The mare that produces an icteric foal does not possess the antigens causing the disease on her erythrocytes, but she can produce antibodies against them if her blood is exposed to them. The lack of the antigens on the red blood cells appears to be a recessive trait. A mare that becomes sensitized is homozygous negative or (--). The stallion, on the other hand, possesses the antigens that react with the antibodies of the mare, and the presence of the antigen is dominant to the lack of it. Thus the stallion can be heterozygous dominant for the genes producing the antigens (/ -) or homozygous dominant (/ /).

Recommendation

The disease has been thoroughly researched and several procedures for preventing its occurrence, or for treating it, have been developed. Before a mating is made, the blood serum of the mare can be mixed with the erythrocytes of the stallion in the laboratory to determine if they are compatible. If they are, the erythrocytes of the stallion will not be destroyed and such a mating should not produce an affected foal. If the blood of the mare and the blood of the stallion are incompatible, however, as shown by the destruction of the erythrocytes of the stallion when they are mixed with the blood serum of the mare, such a mating is not advisable.

Even if the blood of the foal and the blood of its dam are incompatible, the foal is not affected in the uterus. It is not affected until it receives the antibodies from its mother's colostrum.

If a foal that might be susceptible is born, it should not be allowed to nurse its mother until it is determined whether its erythrocytes are compatible with the antibodies in its mother's colostrum. This can be determined by mixing the blood of the foal with the colostrum of the mother. If the test indicates they are compatible, the foal may be allowed to nurse its mother. If the test indicates they are incompatible, certain precautions are necessary. The foal should not receive its mother's milk for at least 48 hours after it is born. After that time the foal no longer absorbs antibodies through its gut into its bloodstream, although there may be some exceptions to this time limit. In the meantime the mare should be hand milked to remove the colostrum from the udder. The foal may then be returned to its mother with much less chance of developing the hemolytic disease.

While it is kept away from its mother, the foal should receive colostrum from a nurse mare or from some other source that does not carry the destructive antibodies. Some also recommend that antibiotics should be administered to the foal during this period.

Once the foal has developed the disease, the treatment recommended is to remove some of the blood of the foal and replace it with a similar amount of blood from a compatible donor. Equipment for a two-way blood exchange transfusion has been developed.

REFERENCES

Archer, R. K. 1961. True haemophilia (haemophilia A) in a Thoroughbred foal. Vet. Rec. 73:338–40.

Bruner, D. W. 1948. Laboratory diagnosis of hemolytic icterus in foals. Cornell Vet. 40:11–16.

Bruner, D. W., and E. R. Doll. 1953. Blood groups in horses (Indian system): Their value in transfusions and neonatal isoerythrolysis. Cornell Vet. 43:217–22.

Bruner, D. W., E. R. Doll, F. E. Hull, and A. S. Kinkaid. 1950. Further studies on hemolytic icterus in foals. Am. J. Vet. Res. 11:22–25.

Bruner, D. W., P. R. Edwards, and E. R. Doll. 1948. Passive immunity in the newborn foal. Cornell Vet. 38:363–66.

Bruner, D. W., F. E. Hull, and E. R. Doll. 1948. The relation of blood factors to icterus in foals. Am. J. Vet. Res. 9:237–42.

Bruner, D. W., F. E. Hull, P. R. Edwards, and E. R. Doll. 1948. Icteric foals. JAVMA 112:440–41.

————. 1948. Twelve jaundiced foal-producing mares. The Blood-Horse 53:24.

Coombs, R. R. A., F. T. Crowhurst, F. T. Day, et al. 1948. Haemolytic disease of newborn foals due to isoimmunization of pregnancy. J. Hyg. 46:403–18.

Cronin, M. T. I. 1950. Haemolytic disease in foals. Irish Vet. J. 4:138–41.

————. 1953. Exchange transfusion in the foal. Vet. Rec. 65:120–23.

————. 1955. Haemolytic disease of newborn foals. Vet. Rec. 67:479–94.

Dimock, W. W., P. R. Edwards, and D. W. Bruner. 1947. Infections observed in equine fetuses and foals. Cornell Vet. 37:89–99.

Doll, E. R. 1952. Observations on the clinical features and pathology of hemolytic icterus on newborn foals. Am. J. Vet. Res. 13:504–8.

————. 1953. Evidence of the production of an anti-isoantibody by foals affected with hemolytic icterus. Cornell Vet. 43:44–51.

Doll, E. R., and F. E. Hull. 1951. Observations on hemolytic icterus of newborn foals. Cornell Vet. 41:14–35.

Doll, E. R., M. G. Richards, M. W. Wallace, and J. T. Bryans. 1952. The influence of an equine fetal tissue vaccine upon haemagglutination activity of mare serums: Its relation to hemolytic icterus of newborn foals. Cornell Vet. 42:495–505.

Farrelly, B. T., and W. C. Miller. 1954. Equine haemolytic disease. Parturient and post-parturient treatment of antibody-positive mares and their foals. Vet. Rec. 66:223–24.

Farrelly, B. T., C. W. A. Belonje, and M. T. I. Cronin. 1950. The technique of exchange transfusion in the newborn foal. Vet. Rec. 62:403–4.

Franks, D. 1962. Horse blood groups and haemolytic disease of the newborn foal. Ann. N. Y. Acad. Sci. 97:235–50.

Howard, F. A., and M. T. I. Cronin. 1955. Colostral transfer of antierythrocyte agglutinins from mare to foal. JAVMA 126:93–94.

Jeffcott, L. B. 1969. Haemolytic disease of the newborn foal. Equine Vet. J. 1:165–70.

Osbaldiston, G. W., J. R. Coffman, and E. C. Stowe. 1969. Equine isoerythrolysis: Clinical pathological observations and transfusion of dam's red blood cells to her foal. Can. J. Comp. Med. 33:310–15.

Parry, H. B., F. T. Day, and R. C. Crowhurst. 1949. Diseases of newborn foals. I. Haemolytic disease due to isoimmunization of pregnancy. Vet. Rec. 61:435–41.

Roberts, E. J., and R. K. Archer. 1966. Current methods for the diagnosis and treatment of haemolytic disease in the foal. Vet. Rec. 79:61–67.

Sanger, V. L., et al. 1964. Hemophilia in a foal. JAVMA 144:259–64.

Stormont, C., et al. 1964. Serology of horse blood groups. Cornell Vet. 54:439–52.

Wallenstein, W. 1949. The Rh factor in Thoroughbreds. M.S.C. Vet. 10:35–38.

Zolinski, J. 1966. Remarks on serological conflict in horses. (Polish) Med. Vet. 22:235–36.

CHAPTER 37

Sensory Organs

ANIRIDIA

Aniridia refers to the condition where the irises of the eyes are missing. In one report the irises of both eyes were entirely lacking at birth, and cataracts developed in the lens 2 months after birth.

Aniridia and the associated cataracts caused reduced vision in most foals. With advancing age most of the affected individuals became totally blind, and while some could see, their vision was abnormal.

Aniridia was noted in 65 of 143 Belgian horses that were the progeny of a single Belgian stallion on the Swedish island Oland. All the dams to which he was mated were normal in vision. The stallion himself was affected but was not completely blind. The condition was not noted in other Belgian horses in the area.

Inheritance

A genetic analysis proved the defect to be in full agreement with the assumption that it was caused by an autosomal dominant gene with complete penetrance. The ratio of affected to normal offspring fit this assumption and normal daughters of this stallion when mated to stallions with normal vision always produced normal offspring.

The stallion's sire and dam apparently had normal eyesight. It appears that the gene arose from a mutation in the gametes of either his sire or dam.

Recommendation

This condition is rare, having been reported only once in the literature. Discarding all defective individuals should eliminate the gene.

REFERENCE

Eriksson, K. 1955. Hereditary aniridia with secondary cataract in horses. Nord. Vet. Med. 7:773–93.

CHAPTER 38

Bones and Joints

MULTIPLE BONE DEFECTS IN SHETLANDS

Fifty ponies were studied from 1961 to 1967. Foals were small compared to normal animals of the same age. The head proportions were normal except the ears, which were usually very stubby. The back was abnormally long and the legs short. The front legs always showed a very short arm and forearm (humerus and radius). Sometimes the junction between the shoulder and the trunk was rather loose, causing a forward and slightly outward position of the point of the shoulder. The foals were often knock-kneed and the front feet showed a toe-out position. In some cases ankylosis of the pastern and pedal joints occurred. Severe malformations of the feet with buckled hooves also occurred. The hind legs were usually less affected but sometimes were cow hocked and sickle hocked.

Inheritance and Recommendation

All affected animals were born of normal-appearing parents. An affected stallion mated with five affected mares produced nine foals showing the malformations. Five apparently normal offspring were produced by mating affected mares with a normal stallion. It was proposed that the condition was caused by an autosomal recessive gene with complete penetrance but with varied expressivity.

Affected individuals and their close relatives should not be used for breeding.

REFERENCE

Hermans, W. A. 1970. A hereditary anomaly in Shetland ponies. Netherland J. Vet. Sci. 3:55–63.

FLEXED FORELEGS

The condition of flexed forelegs has been described at least twice in the literature. The two lower joints of the forelegs were rigidly flexed, with the smaller than normal hooves bent under. The hind legs were normal. Sometimes only one leg was affected. The occurrence of the condition appears to be rare.

Pathophysiology

Foals are born with this condition and are usually so badly crippled that they cannot nurse and have to be destroyed within 2 or 3 days.

Inheritance and Recommendation

The condition is probably recessive, but more work needs to be done to obtain definite proof.

No treatment of the legs is possible. It is best not to remate normal parents that produce such a foal, and if at all possible they should be culled from the herd because they are probably carriers of the recessive gene for this trait.

REFERENCES

Prawochenski, R. 1936. A new lethal factor in the horse (stiff foreleg). J. Hered. 27:410–14.

Pulas, W. L., and F. B. Hutt. 1969. Lethal dominant white in horses. J. Hered. 60:59–63.

LIMB DEFECT

Menzin, an Anglo-Arabian stallion with three quarters of Arabian blood, was used in a Polish stud and sired 26 foals, 8 of which had defects of the forelimbs. One or both forelegs of the defective foals had crooked, immobilized phalanges and underdeveloped shortened hooves resembling small apples. Other hooves were normal. Some of the foals had to be destroyed and others could not nurse without help.

A more severe form of leg defect has been reported in which there is an absence of the foreleg (abracia). The pedigrees of 8 affected individuals were similar and 4 foals were by the same sire.

Both of these conditions are rare in occurrence.

Pathophysiology

A necropsy examination of the limb defect showed an apparent lack of synergistic balance between the flexor and extensor muscles of the limb, with atrophy of muscles higher up on the limb. The absence of a limb probably was due to the failure of cells in the embryo to divide normally and form this part of the body.

Inheritance and Recommendation

The evidence suggests that these are two different defects determined by two different pairs of genes. Both, however, appear to be due to recessive autosomal genes.

Inbreeding should be avoided and affected foals and their parents should not be used for breeding.

REFERENCE

Prawochenski, R. 1936. A new lethal factor in the horse (stiff foreleg). J. Hered. 27:411.

PARROT MOUTH

In one stud, 15.65% of the dams had parrot mouth and the defect occurred in 25.6% of the foals. In another stud, 20.1% of the foals were affected. The condition seemed to be recessive in its mode of inheritance. However, in another study it appeared to be a dominant. Affected individuals should not be used for breeding.

REFERENCES

Bielsanski, W. 1946. The inheritance of the lower jaw (Brachygnathia inferior) in the horse. Przegl. Hodowl 14:24-28; 68-70 (A.B. Abstracts 15:94, 1947).
Hamori, D. 1941. Parrot mouth and hog mouth as inherited deformities. Allatorv. Lapok 64:57 (A.B. Abstract 10:9, 1942).

CHAPTER 39

Neuromuscular System

TORTICOLLIS (Wryneck)

Torticollis is a persistent and involuntary condition in which the cervical muscles are contracted, resulting in a twisted neck and unnatural position of the head. Torticollis is fairly common in horses, but it is usually seen in animals that are several weeks of age and is due to muscular spasms, nerve paralysis, or fracture of the vertebrae. A lethal congenital form of this condition also occurs but is quite rare.

Pathophysiology

Although it is known that the condition is due to the contraction of the neck muscles, the actual physiologic cause for abnormal contraction is not clear.

Inheritance and Recommendation

The congenital form is probably an autosomal recessive trait. In one report, 16 foals showing this trait were inbred and traced to the same stallion. When the condition is observed as the result of an injury, it is probably not due to heredity.

When the condition is congenital, the homozygous recessive individuals are eliminated because it is lethal. Parents of such an individual would be carriers and should be culled and inbreeding avoided.

REFERENCE

Mauderer, H. 1940. Abrachia and torticollis: Lethal factors in horse breeding. Z. Tierz. Zucht. Bld. 51:215 (A.B. Abstracts 10:144).

WOBBLES

American workers have given the name "wobbles" to a syndrome of anomalies that primarily affect the central nervous system. This syndrome appears to be identical to one reported in Europe known as "idiopathic hip lameness." Over 200 cases of wobbles have been reported in Kentucky, and it is found in American Saddlebreds, Standardbreds, and draft breeds. It is seen in horses from 3 months to 3 years of age. It is characterized by an irregularity of the gait, first evident in the movement of the hind legs (ataxic, bilateral incoordination). The symptoms become more severe with the passage of time and may become so severe that affected individuals require help to get to their feet from a recumbent position. Usually affected individuals are able to stand once they are on their feet.

Pathophysiology

From necropsies performed at the Kentucky Agricultural Experiment Station it was found that 15% of the affected individuals showed major gross lesions of the nervous system, 35% minor gross lesions, and 50% exhibited no lesions whatsoever.

Inheritance and Recommendation

Breeding records suggest that wobbles is a recessive trait, but not all wobbler × wobbler matings produce wobbler offspring. This would indicate that the recessive gene for this trait has incomplete penetrance. Foreign workers believe the predisposition for the condition is inherited rather than the condition itself. Some also feel that the condition can result from a number of different processes.

Affected animals should not be kept for breeding and it would be advisable to discard parents of an affected offspring.

REFERENCES

Dimock, W. W. 1950. "Wobbles"—An hereditary disease in horses. J. Hered. 41:319–23.

Dimock, W. W., and B. J. Errington. 1939. Incoordination of Equidae: Wobblers. JAVMA 95:261–67.

Fraser, H. 1966. Two dissimilar types of cerebellar disorder in the horse. Vet. Rec. 78:608–12.

Fraser, H., and A. C. Palmer. 1967. Equine incoordination and wobbler disease of young horses. Vet. Rec. 80:338–55.

Jones, T. C., E. R. Doll, and R. G. Brown. 1954. The pathology of equine incoordination (ataxia or "wobbles" of foals). Proc. Am. Vet. Med. Assoc. 45:139–49.

Matthias, D., O. Dietz, and R. Rechenberger. 1965. Clinical features and pathology of spinal ataxia in foals. Arch. Exp. Vet. Med. 19:43–72.

Montali, R. G., et al. 1974. Spinal ataxia in zebras: Comparison with wobbler syndrome in horses. Vet. Pathol. 111:68–78.

Steel, J. D., J. H. Whittem, and D. R. Hutchins. 1959. Equine sensory ataxia (wobbles). Aust. Vet. J. 35:442–49.

HEREDITARY FOAL ATAXIA

Hereditary foal ataxia has been described only in a German breed of horses, the Oldenberg. Close observation from 1938 to 1948 found 40 male and 30 female foals affected, with 56 of these traced to the same stallion.

Symptoms of the defect appear 3-8 weeks following birth. The affected animals show a failure of muscular coordination or irregular muscular action. Affected individuals stop in the middle of a forward movement, totter, step backward, and go down on their knees and are unable to rise. They also characteristically throw back their heads. Death occurs within 8-14 days after the symptoms first appear.

Pathophysiology

A histopathologic examination of the brain has shown a shrinkage of ganglial cells in certain areas. A ganglion generally refers to neurons containing enlargements of the peripheral nerves. If these cells are located in the central nervous system, perhaps one should substitute "neuron" for "ganglial cells."

Inheritance and Recommendation

The mode of inheritance seems to be a simple autosomal recessive. Affected individuals and their close relatives should not be used for breeding.

REFERENCES

Hippen, F. 1949. Genetical studies of foal ataxia in the Oldenberg breeding area. Dissertation. Tieraerztl. Hochsch., Hanover, Germany.
Koch, P., and H. Fischer. 1950. Hereditary ataxia in the Oldenberg foals. Tieraerztl. Umsch. 5:317-20.
_____. 1951. Oldenberg foal ataxia as a hereditary disease. Tieraerztl. Umsch. 6:158-59.
_____. 1952. Oldenberg foal ataxia as a hereditary disease. Tieraerztl. Umsch. 7:244.

CEREBELLAR HYPOPLASIA AND DEGENERATION

Cerebellar hypoplasia and degeneration are characterized by the inability of the animal to control accurately the range of movement in muscular acts (dysmetria), with overreaching (hypermetria) and, frequently, paddling. Head tremor in a lateral or vertical plane develops in most affected animals and becomes more intense when they are excited. Usually the affected animals stand with their forelegs wide apart. Symptoms of the disease usually appear at 4-6 months of age. The disease seems to be limited to Arab or part Arab horses.

Pathophysiology

Autopsy and histopathologic findings usually show no gross cerebellar atrophy, but histologic studies show a marked reduction in Purkinje cells in the cerebellum, with a mild to moderate thinning of granular and molecular layers.

Inheritance and Recommendation

Heredity appears to be involved, but the mode of inheritance has not been determined. In one study pedigrees of affected foals showed inbreeding with many common ancestors. Since cerebellar hypoplasia and degeneration appear to be limited to the Arab breed, heredity is probably involved. It is also possible that virus infections may be involved and may be predisposing factors in the occurrence of the disease. Cerebellar degeneration has been reported in cats, dogs, cattle, and sheep and appears to be hereditary in some of these species.

Although the condition in horses has not been proved to be hereditary, it would be advisable to cull affected animals and avoid using parents of affected offspring for breeding purposes.

REFERENCES

Baird, J. D., and C. D. Mackenzie. 1974. Cerebellar hypoplasia and degeneration in part Arab horses. Aust. Vet. J. 50:25–28.

Cook, W. R., and A. C. Palmer. 1971. Arab cerebellar disease. Vet. Rec. 88:200.

Dungworth, D. L., and M. E. Fowler. 1966. Cerebellar hypoplasia and degeneration in a foal. Cornell Vet. 56:17–24.

Rooney, J. R. 1963. Equine incoordination. 1. Gross morphology. Cornell Vet. 53:411–22.

Sponseller, M. L. 1967. Equine cerebellar hypoplasia and degeneration. Proc. Am. Assoc. Equine Pract., p. 123.

CHAPTER 40

Digestive System

ATRESIA COLI

Atresia coli is a closure or lack of complete development of the ascending colon in the region of the pelvic flexure. The same condition occurs in other species of livestock as well as in humans.

This condition was observed in the inbred descendants of the Percheron stallion, Superb, imported into Japan from Ohio between 1880 and 1890.

Pathophysiology

Closure of the colon, unless successfully operated upon to alter the obstruction, can result in the death of the individual shortly after birth due to the inability to defecate. In the horse the condition has been reported to be associated with the presence of glioma of the brain, which is a tumor of connective tissue cells of the nervous system. It has also been reported to be associated with hydrocephalus, an abnormal accumulation of fluid in the cranial vault. The genetic association of atresia coli with these two conditions is not clear.

Inheritance and Recommendation

The mode of inheritance seems to be a simple autosomal recessive.

Atresia coli is usually of little importance to the practical breeder. In some species the condition may be caused by virus infections in the mother during the early part of pregnancy, which affects the normal development of the fetus. The same may also be true in horses. In such a case the trait would not be inherited.

246

REFERENCES

Runnells, R. A., W. S. Monlux, and A. W. Monlux. 1960. Principles of Veterinary Pathology. Ames: Iowa State Univ. Press.

Wriedt, C. 1926. As reported by F. A. E. Crew, and A. D. Buchanan Smith. The genetics of the horse. Bibliog. Genetica 6:123–70.

Yamane, J. 1927. As reported by J. N. Eaton, 1937. Summary of lethal characters in animals and man. J. Hered. 28:324–26.

CHAPTER 41

Urogenital System

TWINNING

Some may not consider twinning in horses as a defect but in many cases it is more serious than a disease. The reason for this is that many twin pregnancies result in abortions usually between 7 and 9 months of pregnancy. Even when carried to near term, twins may cause dystocia, which often results in the death of the young and sometimes in the death or eventual destruction of the dam. Although twinning probably should not be classed among the lethals, it is an important source of economic loss to the horse breeder.

American data show a 1.72% twinning rate in Belgians and a 4.37% twinning rate in Percherons. In Europe, a study of 39,436 animals of the Rhenish breed found a twinning rate of 1.12%. In one stud, percentages for twinning were 2.34%, 3.13%, and 5.34% for three different family groups.

Pathophysiology

Twinning in horses is mostly due to the ovulation of two or more eggs during a single estrous period. The usual ovulation in mares produces a single ovum, but an overproduction of follicle-stimulating hormone (FSH) and luteinizing hormone (LH) or a greater response of the ovary to the stimulation of the gonadotrophic hormones may be responsible for more than one egg being produced by the ovary in a given heat period.

Identical twins resulting from the division of a single fertilized egg may also occur in horses. The percentage of identical twins in horses is not definitely known. About 5%–8% of all twins in cattle are identical and probably a similar percentage could be expected in horses.

Inheritance and Recommendation

Research leaves little doubt that twinning is inherited because it occurs much more frequently in some families than others. Some work suggests that twinning in horses is due to a single recessive gene, but it is also possible that more than one pair of genes (polygenes) are involved. Environmental factors such as a high level of nutrition and a productive age, neither young or old, may also be predisposing factors.

Some horse breeders discriminate against mares or family lines that produce twins, since twinning is inherited and is of economic importance due to the high death losses in twin foals. Twinning probably does not occur often enough to warrant selection against it. Some practitioners abort twin foals or cause their resorption early in fetal life when they are detected.

REFERENCES

Blakeslee, L. H., and R. S. Hudson. 1942. Twinning in horses. J. Anim. Sci. 1:155.
Robertson, W. R. B. 1917. A mule and horse as twins and the inheritance of twinning. Kansas Univ. Sci. Bull. 10:293.
Wriedt, C. 1928. Inheritance of twins in horses. Zuchtungskunde 3:455.

CRYPTORCHIDISM

The failure of the testicles to descend into the scrotum is known as cryptorchidism and occurs in many species of animals. The failure of one testicle to descend into the scrotum is a unilateral cryptorchid. The failure of both testicles to descend is a bilateral cryptorchid.

Castration normally removes both testicles, but in the cryptorchid the testicle or testicles in the body cavity are not removed. A special type of operation would be required to remove the testicle from the body cavity. Such an operation is costly and time-consuming and is usually not practical. Cryptorchidism occurs frequently in horses. Unilateral cryptorchidism when one testicle is removed and the other remains in the body cavity is responsible for a "ridgling," a term often used by horsebreeders to describe cryptorchidism. It is a very undesirable trait and is avoided by those who use horses for riding or working.

Pathophysiology

A bilateral cryptorchid horse is sterile because the testicles cannot produce spermatozoa when they are maintained at the normal body temperature. The scrotum normally maintains a temperature several degrees below the temperature of the body, which allows sperm production. Even though a bilateral cryptorchid is sterile, he has all the sex drive and sexual characteristics of the intact male, or stallion, because he produces the male hormone testosterone.

The unilateral cryptorchid normally is fertile because one testicle has descended to the scrotum and produces sperm at that temperature. The removal of one testicle during castration still leaves one testicle in the body cavity that continues to produce the male hormone testosterone. Such males, although sterile, have all the outward characteristics of stallions. They are avoided in working cattle or where large groups of horses are run together in a herd or remuda. Their tendency to fight, bite, and kick may injure other horses in the group.

Inheritance and Recommendation

The mode of inheritance of cryptorchidism in horses is not clear, but inheritance does seem to be involved. Evidence of the genetic nature of this trait is provided by information from the Hungarian National Stud Farm which recorded two instances in which bilateral or unilateral cryptorchidism was transmitted through two or three generations. In another stud where a monorchid stallion was used for breeding, eight of his forty sons were cryptorchids (six unilateral and two bilateral). His fertility also was only 23.2% as compared to 53% for the whole stud. One of his sons produced ten male offspring of which one was a cryptorchid and another showed a delay of the descent of the testicles into the scrotum. The mode of inheritance was considered to be a dominant.

No males that are unilateral cryptorchids should be retained for breeding purposes, nor should mares producing a cryptorchid son be used for breeding.

REFERENCES

Basrur, P. L., et al. 1969. An equine intersex with unilateral gonadal agenesis. Can. J. Comp. Med. 33:297–306.

Bergin, W. C., et al. 1970. A developmental concept of equine cryptorchidism. Biol. Reprod. 3:82–92.

Brook, D. 1969. Equine cryptorchidism. Vet. Rec. 84:258–59.

Flechsig, J. 1950. Hereditary cryptorchidism in a depot stallion. Tierzucht. 4:208.

_____. 1952. Unilateral abdominal cryptorchidism in a depot stallion, and its genetical analysis. Dissertation. Freie University, Berlin. Abstract in Berl. Munch. Tieraerztl. Wochenschr. 65:75–76.

Frye, J. 1968. The operational procedure during the castration of stallions with abdominal cryptorchidism. (Polish, English summary.) Med. Vet. 24:270–72.

Hamori, D. 1940. Data on the heredity of equine cryptorchidism. Allatorv. Lapok 63:130–31.

Lowe, J. E., et al. 1969. Castration of abdominal cryptorchid horses by a paramedian laparotomy approach. Cornell Vet. 59:121–26.

O'Connor, J. P. 1969. Some aspects of cryptorchidism in the horse (Abstract only). Vet. Rec. 85:145.

_____. 1971. Rectal examination of the cryptorchid horse. Irish Vet. J. 25:129–31.

INTERSEXUALITY

Intersexuality in horses has been reported in the literature since 1687. Many of the early reports, however, did not distinguish between cryptorchids and intersexes. More recently chromosome studies have been reported in intersex horses. The degree of intersexuality varies from one extreme to another. Some intersexes have the outward appearance of a stallion but the external genitalia usually include a vulva and a rudimentary or well-developed penis emerging from the skin folds between the hind legs at a position approximately midway between the normal male and the female anogenital distances. Testicles are sometimes present in the abdomen and one instance was reported where one testicle had descended into the scrotum.

Pathophysiology

Cultures from peripheral leukocytes, or from the descended testicle in one case, indicate a chromosome abnormality. In one case a drumstick (type) was present on the neutrophils, indicating a female genotype and possibly an XXY chromosome complement. A further study of this case, however, indicated a whole body chimerism resulting from the double fertilization of a single egg or the fusion of two blastocysts. Another case revealed a 64 XX/65 XXY mosaicism in an intersex, while a third case was reported as an XXXY individual with the normal complement of autosomes.

Inheritance and Recommendation

Although chromosome abnormalities are involved in some intersexes, no reports indicate intersexuality is inherited. It is more likely due to accidental abnormalities involving the segregation of chromosomes in the gametes during gametogenesis. Double fertilization of a single ovum or the union of two blastocysts may also occur.

Since the condition is rare and not hereditary, no recommendations appear to be justified.

REFERENCES

Basrur, P. K., H. Kanagawa, and J. P. W. Gilman. 1969. An equine intersex with unilateral gonadal agenesis. Can. J. Comp. Med. 33:297–306.

Basrur, P. K., H. Kanagawa, and L. Podliachouk. 1970. Further studies on the cell populations of an intersex horse. Can. J. Comp. Med. 34:294–97.

Bouters, R., M. Vandeplassche, and A. De Moor. 1972. An intersex (male pseudohermaphrodite) horse with 64XX/65XXY mosaicism. Equine Vet. J. 4:150–53.

Dunn, H. O., J. T. Vaughan, and K. McEntee. 1974. Bilaterally cryptorchid stallion with a female karyotype. Cornell Vet. 64:265–75.

Gerneke, W. H., and R. I. Coubrough. 1970. Intersexuality in the horse. Onderstepoort J. Vet. Res. 37:211–16.

Gluhovschi, N., M. Bistriceano, A. Suciol, and M. Bratu. 1970. A case of intersexuality in the horse with type 2A-XXXY chromosome formula. Br. Vet. J. 126:522–25.

ANEUPLOIDY

Aneuploidy is a chromosome abnormality in which there are one or more chromosomes or one or less chromosomes in the body cells than normal. This is distinguished from polyploidy in which entire sets of chromosomes (3n, 4n, etc.) are duplicated.

The chromosome complement of a 12-year-old infertile thoroughbred mare was found to consist of 63 rather than the normal 64 chromosomes. Normal X chromosomes were not identified, but a small subterminal chromosome was present, which was absent in the normal chromosome complement. The small, unidentified chromosome may have resulted from the breakage and rearrangement of the X chromosome during gametogenesis in the dam. A causal relationship seemed to exist between the mare's infertility and the condition of aneuploidy.

REFERENCE

Payne, H. W., K. Ellsworth, and A. DeGroot. 1968. Aneuploidy in an infertile mare. JAVMA 153:1293-99.

CHAPTER 42

Skin

CURLY COAT

In a study in Europe it was found that about 3% of Lakai horses have a curly coat. Curly × curly matings gave 46 curly to 13 normal offspring. Curly × normal gave 17 curly to 20 normal offspring. No sex linkage was indicated and coat color was not related to a curly coat. About one-third of the curly offspring from curly parents showed a marked degree of curliness at birth and it was proposed that these were homozygotes. The data indicated that in this breed of horses the trait was recessive.

A study of curly coat in Percherons in the United States also indicated the trait was recessive. Sixteen mares bred to a son of the half brother of these mares' sire produced 37 smooth and 5 curly foals.

The curly coat in horses did not seem to be undesirable from the standpoint of type and performance.

REFERENCES

Blakeslee, L. H., R. S. Hudson, and H. R. Hunt. 1943. Curly coat in horses. J. Hered. 34:115–18.
Shchekin, V. A., and V. V. Kalaev. 1940. Inheritance of curliness in the horse. C. R. (Dokl.) Acad. Sci. U.R. ss, N.S. 26:262–63 (A.B. Abstracts 9:7,1941).

EPITHELIOGENESIS IMPERFECTA (HAIRLESSNESS)

Skin and hair defects have been reported in many species of animals, including horses. Affected foals are born alive but seldom survive for more than a few days. One report cites 33 cases of this condition over a

22-year period mostly in cold-blooded foals. It has occurred in scattered instances in many parts of the world but is relatively rare.

Pathophysiology

In affected foals the hair coat is abnormal with patches on the legs having no hair, and in these areas the skin resembles a tanned hide. Sometimes a hoof is missing or imperfectly attached to the skin.

Inheritance and Recommendation

An autosomal recessive gene mode of inheritance is indicated.

Discard all affected individuals as well as their parents and avoid inbreeding.

REFERENCE

Butz, H., and H. Meyer. 1957. Epitheliogenesis imperfecta in foals. Dtsch. Tieraerztl. Wochenschr. 64:555–59.

CHAPTER 43

Other Structures

HERNIA

Both umbilical and inguinal hernias have been reported in horses. The occurrence of these hernias in horses as listed by case records from 12 United States and Canadian Veterinary College Hospital clinics is shown in Table 43.1.

Table 43.1. Occurrence of umbilical and inguinal hernias in horses

Breed or Type	Umbilical Hernias	Inguinal Hernias	Total of All Horses Checked
Arabian	11	10	5,188
Draft horses & mules	8	3	11,590
Ponies (Shetland & Welch)	2	0	3,441
Quarter horses	147	9	21,188
Standardbred	21	15	7,453
Thoroughbreds	49	5	9,195
Other saddle horses	55	29	15,201

Males had more inguinal hernias $(P < .01)$ and females more umbilical hernias $(P < .05)$.

In one study of 94 foals from 3 affected stallions, 79 were born with umbilical, 11 with scrotal (5 were also cryptorchid), and 2 with inguinal hernias while 2 had a fistula of the umbilical cord and urachus. In another study of the inheritance of inguinal hernia in the horse, it was reported that two recessive factors were involved, one causing unusual width of the ring and the other a slight stretching of the sac of the tunica vaginalis.

Even though reports are not always specific on the inheritance of hernias, they do indicate that inheritance is involved. Therefore, it is recommended that breeding stock with any form of hernia should not be retained for breeding.

REFERENCES

Aurich, R. 1959. A contribution to the inheritance of umbilical hernia in the horse. Berl. Munch. Tieraerztl. Wochenschr. 72:420–23 (A.B. Abstracts 28:110, 1960).

Hamori, D. 1940. Inheritance of the tendency to hernia in horses. Allatoru Lapok 63:136 (A.B. Abstracts 10:9, 1942).

Hayes, H. M. 1974. Congenital umbilical and inguinal hernias in cattle, horses, swine, dogs, and cats: Risk by breed and sex among hospital patients. Am. J. Vet. Res. 35:839–42.

Schlaak, F. 1941. Investigations on the inheritance of umbilical hernia in a horse breeding region. Z. Tierz. Zuchtbiol. 52:298 (A.B. Abstracts 10:211, 1942).

Wagner, H. 1941. Contribution to the inheritance of inguinal hernia in the horse. Berl. Munch. Tieraerztl. Wochenschr., pp. 386–88 (A.B. Abstracts 10:145, 1942).

Wille, H. 1945. Is inguinal hernia hereditary in the horse? Norsk. Vet. Tidsskr. 57:332 (A.B. Abstracts 15:10, 1947).

LARYNGEAL HEMIPLEGIA (ROARING)

Roaring refers to the noise made by horses when they take air into their lungs. Such horses are sometimes referred to as being "thick in the wind." The condition has often been described in horses all over the world.

Roaring probably involves the nervous system and is seen in all types of horses, but in the United States it affects mostly the racing breeds. Some have reported the condition as primary in which it occurs without apparent cause, and secondary in which it occurs following an infectious disease or during old age.

In addition to true roaring, several other abnormalities cause similar symptoms. One of these may be described as intermittent spasms of the larynx, and another is an unnatural type of respiration in which the timing of breathing appears to be upset. Care must be taken not to mistake these for roaring per se.

Pathophysiology

The picture concerning this condition is quite confused. Veterinarians consider true roaring as a complete or partial unilateral or bilateral paralysis of the nerve that innervates the intrinsic muscles of the larynx.

Inheritance and Recommendation

Reports are not in full agreement on the mode of inheritance of this trait, although there is considerable evidence to suggest that it does have a genetic base. Some studies suggest that it is due to a single autosomal dominant gene. Others do not support this mode of inheritance although there does seem to be a genetic base. Perhaps the right environmental conditions are necessary for the full expression of the trait in individuals possessing the genes responsible for the defect.

Although the actual mode of inheritance has not been determined, there is little doubt that the tendency toward roaring is inherited. The practical breeder, therefore, should strongly select against individuals showing this particular defect, and none should be used for breeding purposes.

REFERENCES

Oppermann, T., and M. Oppermann. 1943. Is roaring a hereditary defect? Derl. Munch. Tieraerztl. Wochenschr. and Wien. Tieraerztl. Mschr., p. 346 (A.B. Abstract 13:72).

Runciman, B. 1941. Roaring and whistling in Thoroughbred horses. Vet. Rec. 53:37-38.

Robb, W. 1936. Hereditary diseases. Vet. Rec. 48:811-15.

Schaper, U. 1939. On the inheritance of roaring in the horse. Dtsch. Tieraerztl. 47:385 (A.B. Abstracts 8, 105, 1940).

Weiss, K. 1940. On the inheritance of roaring with special reference to the study of blood lines. Z. Veterinark 52:16-17.

Wharam, S. 1941. Roaring and whistling in Thoroughbred horses. Vet. Rec. 53:91.

CRIBBING AND WINDSUCKING

Cribbing and windsucking are closely associated. Cribbing is a condition in which affected animals grasp something (fence boards or mangers) with their teeth, chew, arch their necks, and make swallowing motions. They may also set their teeth against an object while sucking in air. Windsuckers perform all these same motions in addition to swallowing large volumes of air. The condition may develop any time from weaning until an animal becomes an adult. These afflictions result in loss of condition and injury to the teeth. Such horses are more subject to colic.

These conditions are widespread, especially in Thoroughbreds, American Saddlebred, and Standardbred horses. It is believed to affect about 5% of the adult population.

Pathophysiology

The physiology of cribbing and windsucking is not clear. It may develop because of a lack of some nutrient in the diet or because of boredom due to being tied in the same stall for many hours of the day. The latter seems to be the most logical cause and therefore may be psychological.

Inheritance and Recommendation

Some evidence suggests an autosomal recessive type of inheritance. A strap buckled around the neck helps prevent this vice. An operation has been developed that is often successful but somewhat dangerous. Affected animals should not be kept for breeding.

REFERENCES

Steele, D. G. 1958. The elements of genetics. Stud Managers Handbook. Stud Managers Course, Lexington, Kentucky, pp. 200–206.

―――. 1959. Crib biting and wind sucking of the Thoroughbred. Ky. Farm & Home Sci. 5(4):3, 8.

LETHAL DOMINANT WHITE

Several different kinds of white horses are known and they usually are referred to as albinos. However, it has been suggested that no true albinos with a white coat and pink eyes have ever been seen. At least, most albino horses, if not all, have colored eyes and are referred to as pseudo (false) albinos.

Cremellos are a pale cream color or almost white with a pinkish skin and blue eyes. They are basically colored horses, which also are homozygous for the dilution gene (D) or are of genotype (DD). One dilution gene (D) produces the palomino color when present with the chestnut or sorrel genes (bb).

Another kind of white in horses is one in which the foal is fully colored at birth but has a progressively increased number of white hairs with age until they become practically white. This kind of white has been referred to as progressive silvering or gray.

Dominant white in horses is different from the two kinds of white previously mentioned. Dominant white foals are white at birth but their eyes are either blue or some other color such as brown or hazel. Their skin is pink although dark spots occur in the hooves and they sometimes have dark streaks.

All three types of white occur quite frequently and may be mistaken for the same white color unless the ancestors and progeny are studied closely. The cremello white comes from ancestors in which palominos occur, whereas the gray color can be distinguished from the dominant white because the foals are colored at birth but turn gray or white with age.

Pathophysiology

When dominant white horses are mated, about one-fourth of the developing individuals are not viable. The actual time of the death of the fetus has not been determined, but it occurs sometime before birth and probably early in gestation.

Inheritance and Recommendation

The dominant white color is due to the dominant white gene (W), which is epistatic to all color genes. Breeding tests show that all white individuals of breeding age are heterozygous (genotype Ww), because when mated they produce about 2 white to 1 colored offspring. This has led to the conclusion that the homozygous white genotype (WW) is lethal and never seen, which is further verified by the fact that all white individuals appear to be heterozygous.

Nothing can be done to prevent the death of the homozygous white (WW) individuals. The mating of white horses would result in a 25% death loss, but these losses may be early enough in pregnancy that they would result only in delayed foaling in some mares. If the breeder is trying to produce purebreeding white horses, this would be impossible if all dominant white horses are heterozygous. Mating white with white would result in an average of two-thirds of the foals being white and one-third colored, whereas white mated with colored would give a ratio of 1 white to 1 colored, on the average.

REFERENCES

Berge, S. 1963. Hestefargenes genetikk. Tidsskr. f. Det Norske Landbruk. 70:359–410.
Castle, W. E. 1954. Coat color inheritance in horses and in other mammals. Genetics 39:35–44.
Pulos, W. L., and F. B. Hutt. 1969. Lethal dominant white in horses. J. Hered. 60:59–63.
Wriedt, C. 1924. Vererbungsfaktoren bei weissen Pierden im Gestud Friedriksborg. Zeit. Tierzucht. u. Zuchtungsbiol. 1:231–42.

Section B:

DEFECTS WITH A POSSIBLE GENETIC BASE

CHAPTER 44

Sensory Organs

EYE DEFECT

A stallion exhibited a maldevelopment of the iris and secondary progressive opacity of the lens of the eye. The majority of his offspring showed the same condition in varying degrees. A dominant gene appeared to be the cause.

Affected individuals should not be used for breeding.

REFERENCE

Eriksson, T., and H. Sandstedt. 1938. Hereditary malformation of the iris and ciliary body with secondary cataract in the horse. Svensk VeTidskr. 43:11–14.

CHAPTER 45

Bones and Joints

MULTIPLE EXOSTOSIS

Multiple exostosis is a bone disease in which there are numerous abnormal projections (spurs) of the bones. The cortex and medulla of the bony projections are continuous with that of the bones from which they arise. Exostosis occurs in the long bones, ribs, and the pelvic bones.

The condition was described in four quarter horses. Two fillies sired by the same stallion with the defect were also defective.

Inheritance and Recommendation

If inherited, the mode of inheritance has not been established, but it is recommended that affected individuals not be used for breeding.

REFERENCES

Morgan, J. P., W. D. Carlson, and O. R. Adams. 1962. Hereditary multiple exostosis in the horse. JAVMA 140:1320–22.

Shupe, J. L., et al. 1970. Multiple exostosis in horses. Mod. Vet. Pract. 51:34–36.

PATELLA LUXATION (Congenital)

Congenital lateral luxation of the patella (out of joint, dislocation) has been reported in both horses and ponies. Its occurrence is rare, but there are some indications it may be inherited. The mode of inheritance is unknown.

REFERENCES

Finocchio, E. J., and M. M. Guffy. 1970. Congenital patellar ectopia in a foal. JAVMA 156:222–23.

Hickman, J., and R. G. Walker. 1964. Upward retention of the patella in the horse. Vet. Rec. 76:1198–99.

Rathor, S. S. 1968. Clinical aspects of functional disorders of the equine and bovine femoro-patellar articulation with some remarks on its biomechanics. Drukkerj, Joeljen Kos, Utrecht.

Rooney, J. R., C. W. Raker, and K. J. Harmany. 1971. Congenital lateral luxation of the patella in the horse. Cornell Vet. 61:670–73.

CHAPTER 46

Neuromuscular System

STRINGHALT

Stringhalt is an excessive flexing of the hind legs of the horse. It has been claimed to be inherited through the male line, but the mode of inheritance has not been determined

REFERENCE

Hitenkou, G. G. 1941. Stringhalt in horses and its inheritance. Vestn Seljskashov. Nauki Zivotn, No. 2, 64–76 (A.B. Abstacts 14:137, 1946).

CHAPTER 47

Endocrine and Metabolic Systems

DIABETES MELLITUS

Diabetes mellitus is very rare in horses, but one case was described in the Colorado State University clinic. A 23-year-old mare weighing about 1,000 pounds and of mixed breeding was found to have lipemia, hypercholesterolemia, increased serum transaminase concentration, and hyperglycemia. The mare had a tumor of the pituitary gland. While a relationship between the abnormal pituitary and diabetes mellitus may be involved, a causal relationship has not been definitely established. No evidence was found to indicate that the condition was inherited.

REFERENCE

Tasker, J. B., C. E. Whiteman, and B. R. Marlin. 1966. Diabetes mellitus in the horse. JAVMA 149:393–99.

INDEX